T0201946

The Language of Medicine

The Language of Medicine

Abraham Fuks, MD, CM

Professor of Medicine, McGill University

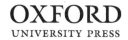

OXFORD
UNIVERSITY PRESS

OXFORD
UNIVERSITY PRESS

Oxford University Press is a department of the University of Oxford. It furthers
the University's objective of excellence in research, scholarship, and education
by publishing worldwide. Oxford is a registered trade mark of Oxford University
Press in the UK and certain other countries.

Published in the United States of America by Oxford University Press
198 Madison Avenue, New York, NY 10016, United States of America.

© Oxford University Press 2021

All rights reserved. No part of this publication may be reproduced, stored in
a retrieval system, or transmitted, in any form or by any means, without the
prior permission in writing of Oxford University Press, or as expressly permitted
by law, by license, or under terms agreed with the appropriate reproduction
rights organization. Inquiries concerning reproduction outside the scope of the
above should be sent to the Rights Department, Oxford University Press, at the
address above.

You must not circulate this work in any other form
and you must impose this same condition on any acquirer.

Library of Congress Cataloging-in-Publication Data
Names: Fuks, Abraham, author.
Title: The language of medicine / Abraham Fuks.
Description: New York, NY : Oxford University Press, [2021] |
Includes bibliographical references and index.
Identifiers: LCCN 2021016414 (print) | LCCN 2021016415 (ebook) |
ISBN 9780190944834 (paperback) | ISBN 9780190944858 (epub) |
ISBN 9780190944865 (online)
Subjects: MESH: Physician-Patient Relations | Language |
Attitude of Health Personnel
Classification: LCC R727.3 (print) | LCC R727.3 (ebook) |
NLM W 62 | DDC 610.69/6—dc23
LC record available at https://lccn.loc.gov/2021016414
LC ebook record available at https://lccn.loc.gov/2021016415

DOI: 10.1093/med/9780190944834.001.0001

This material is not intended to be, and should not be considered, a substitute for medical or other
professional advice. Treatment for the conditions described in this material is highly dependent on the
individual circumstances. And, while this material is designed to offer accurate information with respect
to the subject matter covered and to be current as of the time it was written, research and knowledge about
medical and health issues is constantly evolving and dose schedules for medications are being revised
continually, with new side effects recognized and accounted for regularly. Readers must therefore always
check the product information and clinical procedures with the most up-to-date published product
information and data sheets provided by the manufacturers and the most recent codes of conduct and
safety regulation. The publisher and the authors make no representations or warranties to readers, express
or implied, as to the accuracy or completeness of this material. Without limiting the foregoing, the
publisher and the authors make no representations or warranties as to the accuracy or efficacy of the drug
dosages mentioned in the material. The authors and the publisher do not accept, and expressly disclaim,
any responsibility for any liability, loss, or risk that may be claimed or incurred as a consequence of the use
and/or application of any of the contents of this material.

3 5 7 9 8 6 4 2

Printed by Marquis, Canada

Dedicated
to
Sacvan Bercovitch z"l
1933–2014
Colleague, Mentor, and Friend

Contents

Introduction   ix

I. LANGUAGE IN CONTEXT

1. The Lens of Language   3

2. From Words to "Making Up People"   17

3. The Nature of Metaphor   33

II. THE MILITARY METAPHORS OF MEDICINE

4. The Militarized Arena of Medicine   49

5. Sources of the Military Metaphors of Medicine   63

6. Consequences of the Verbal Wars   77

7. Resilience of Military Metaphors   95

III. FRAMES AND CHOICES

8. In Other Words   109

9. Listening   123

10. A Pharmacology of Words   139

IV. HEALING THE LANGUAGE AND THE LANGUAGE OF HEALING

11. The Physician–Patient Relationship   161

12. Healing Metaphors   179

Afterword   193
Notes   197
Bibliography   207
Index   217

Introduction

Health and illness are of compelling interest to us all. Health care is a recurrent theme in our daily newspapers and blogs and is increasingly entwined with big business, shrinking budgets, partisan politics, and robotic high technology. The successes of modern medicine and the health professions in general are evident. Trauma care, organ transplants, intensive care units, coronary stents, and minimally invasive surgery have extended life expectancy and improved the quality of many lives. Public health measures—for example, high rates of vaccination of children throughout the world—have virtually eliminated serious viral diseases of childhood in many countries, and greater access to midwives and maternal nutrition has decreased perinatal mortality. Another remarkable example is the development and deployment of a vaccine to prevent HPV (human papillomavirus) infections that will dramatically reduce the incidence of cervical cancer in the very near future. A more recent one is the extraordinarily rapid development of an effective vaccine for SARS-Cov-2.

Amidst these burgeoning benefits, we are beset by announcements of a crisis in medicine that is one of a set of puzzling paradoxes. By any number of criteria, contemporary medicine is doing a fine job, yet people everywhere seem disgruntled with the state of health care. Patients generally appreciate their own physicians, yet many have low regard for the medical profession as a whole. What patients seek is flexible and ready access to their physicians and continuity of care. Above all, they want a physician who will listen to them. A clinician who is present to and for the patient, and whose engagement and commitment are made clear in attentiveness and listening. Perversely, the length of the typical medical interaction has shortened substantially, and the patient community has increasingly turned to the Internet to unearth what is often substandard and risky advice. Patients' involvement in their own care can make an important contribution, but it cannot serve as a substitute for thoughtful encounters with health care professionals. Even as practicing physicians complain about third-party interference in medical decision-making, young graduates, concerned with the quality of their own lives, choose non-traditional practices in clinics with fixed hours and interchangeable doctors. The unintended consequences of such choices are a mode of work and trajectory of care that span seconds and minutes rather than months and years and undermine the development of a long-term clinical relationship. We may have arrived at an era of stroboscopic medicine. Patients experience brief episodes of disjointed care in walk-in clinics and urgent care centers. While offering convenient access, such services cannot offer the relational care that patients generally seek.

The structural stresses in the health care system are reflected in the non-ending search by medicine for new models of care. Thus, we have witnessed the advent, with great fanfare, of person-, patient-, and client-centered care. We now have targeted care, personalized medicine, precision medicine, and genetic prognostication. It is often not clear whether such trumpeted innovations ever move beyond the rhetorical phase to actual implementation. These seemingly new, yet often poorly defined, proposals reflect an underlying confusion and instability in the conceptual frameworks of health care.

New technologies have also introduced an array of unintended consequences. Electronic health records prevent many errors in prescriptions and improve the accessibility of hospital and clinic files. Paradoxically, however, the desktop computers that make this possible have become competitors for the physician's attention that is directed to the machine and away from the patient in the room. Patients express discomfort when the doctor's eyes are turned to the screen rather than the person's face and the physician's hands are on a keyboard rather than a stethoscope. The same computers enable the examination of thousands of medical records and millions of data points so that clinical scientists can spot trends and generate hypotheses that may lead to better care. Yet, the nascent field of artificial intelligence is often viewed by the public with some concern and even trepidation. This may in part be the result of the mystery that surrounds neural networks; even the experts are not always certain how this software arrives at its conclusions. However, this fear may also be a result of the sociocultural images evoked by the infelicitous phrase, artificial intelligence, that leads to the implicit question: Will robots replace doctors?

Another unanticipated result of technologies for noninvasive imaging are the incidental and irrelevant findings by powerful imaging machines that lead to needless follow-ups and sometimes risky interventions. The phenomenon of so-called incidentalomas has brought new meaning to the word *serendipity*, though without its traditionally happy connotations. These CAT scanners and MRI magnets permit marvelous feats of diagnosis but do their work by sending beams through patients' bodies without, paradoxically, illuminating the persons who brought their troubles to their physicians in the first place. The physician can once again inspect results on a computer screen without addressing the patient. Finally, the most recent headlines pointing to leaders in biomedicine who failed to reveal serious conflicts of interest have also, and quite understandably, undermined the trust of a vulnerable public. These social, economic, and political forces have resulted in enormous strains on the doctor–patient relationship that is the basis of diagnosis, treatment, and care.

Clinical medicine is enacted in the clinic and hospital, and the participants are the patient and physician. The relationship between these two persons is mediated through language and the interactions between them enable understanding and healing. This dyadic interplay is the locus of the practice of medicine and all the various forces and pressures alluded to previously impinge directly or indirectly on this focal point that is the clinical relationship.

This book is grounded in the notion that the language used by physicians and patients in their interactions, and the words, metaphors, and concepts that form the societal discourse within and about medicine and health care reflect and inflect clinical care. The words we choose and use in any social and personal interaction shape the messages we convey and are the means of transferring information. Words reflect the emotional content of our statements and reveal the states of mind of the interlocutors. Moreover, the words we have and use have the power to shape our views of the world and the people and objects within it. Words frame and reshape our thoughts, since language not only names the world in which we live, it also acts to constitute our reality—to create it and mold it. Clinical interactions are particularly sensitive to the words and linguistic frames that are employed by the participants to communicate concerns, illuminate meanings, and achieve their goals. The stakes are high for both patient and physician and the issues at hand are fraught with significance and tension. Patients listen with great intensity to the words of the physician whose diagnostic judgments and prophetic prognostications may turn daily lives topsy-turvy. Furthermore, patients are trying to decipher the implicit meanings and subtexts beneath the surface of the medical discourse to understand the implications for their health and well-being. And, of course, they wish also to grasp the emotional resonances of the doctors' words to calibrate the seriousness of the situation and as metrics of their caregivers' engagement and concern for their plight.

The first part of the book, Language in Context, begins with a description of clinical practice as seen through the lens of language. The relationship between patient and caregiver is mediated by language with impact. Words are used by the patient to narrate the story of the illness and to convey its meaning and import for that person. In turn, the doctor's apprehension of the narrative and its transformation into the story in the medical chart are both linguistic acts. The words chosen by these interlocutors in the clinical arena may reveal bias, signal concern, herald misfortune, or support healing. Words are hardly neutral modes of communication. They convey and reveal emotion and influence the listener's state of mind. Putting words to things may bring them to our attention and make certain ideas apparent to us. Language influences our thoughts and can enhance or diminish the relevance of both the concrete and the metaphysical by shaping the frames of our perception. In Chapter 2, we explore the idea that language organizes our "house of being" and how that concept is especially relevant to an analysis of clinical care.

Metaphors occur approximately every twenty-five words in daily spoken and written language. They create new understandings by carrying meanings from one domain to another and thereby shift attention toward certain aspects of a thing or idea and away from others. Metaphors open new doors while closing others and reshape our views of the world we inhabit. To set the scene for the major themes of the book, we therefore describe metaphors in Chapter 3: their prevalence, impact, and role in language and discourse.

Part II, The Military Metaphors of Medicine, comprises four chapters that elaborate and dissect a major thread of this work, namely, that the most common metaphor of the language of medicine invokes wars, fights, and enemies—to wit, the war on cancer, the fight to eradicate polio, the campaign against opioid addiction. We fight disease under doctors' orders, targeting magic bullets with precision medicine. Drug companies develop the therapeutic armamentarium and patients may be survivors. We begin with the most prevalent of this class of metaphors and trace its origins through the history of medicine in Chapters 4 and 5. A number of hypotheses have been proposed on the genesis of such linguistic tropes with examples as far back as the early seventeenth century. Chapters 6 and 7 deal with the variations of the war or military metaphor by attending to the protagonists, the enemies, and the allies. Who is fighting whom and why? Who are the winners and losers? While these may appear to be innocent stylistic choices, in actuality these verbal wars have unfortunate consequences. For example, when the surgeon is armed to extirpate a tumor, the patient becomes the passive field of battle and suffers collateral damage. Or, a diagnostic search for the reified disease becomes the object of the physician's attention and the patient is transformed from an ill person to a vessel bearing the invader. At the same time, the ubiquity of such metaphors requires an explanation. If they are deleterious to our understanding of medical care, if not to care itself, why are they so prevalent and pervasive? What accounts for their resilience despite their linguistic side effects? These questions are followed by a broader appreciation of the effects of the military metaphor in reframing the relationship between doctor and patient. Their interaction becomes reshaped and undermined by these tropes whose influence may alter the attitude of physicians to their craft. Doctors learn to deal with disease and are blinded to illness; diagnosis becomes a search for an offending agent or invader rather than an understanding of the patient's life story and the reasons for seeking medical care; preventive medicine is rendered as border walls blocking foreign viruses; and public health is reshaped as epidemiological announcements of high states of red alert against influenza or drug addiction. All such consequences of the language we use in and about medicine are hardly conducive to the type of clinical care to which we aspire in which ailing patients encounter attentive physicians who choose to understand the needs, goals, and implicit meanings of those who seek care, in order to provide healing.

Part III, Frames and Choices, explores specific aspects of clinical practice. If military metaphors are not good for our health, what other tropes can we envisage? Perhaps there are alternative framings of disease and illness that may better serve patients and their caregivers. For example, illness as a journey permits the caregiver to serve as guide or navigator and offers the ill person an option of being the driver or engaged passenger, depending on that individual's inclination. It also provides a continuing narrative of the trip that flows from and perhaps back to the antecedent state of health. From the Western medical canon, we can recall and recover constructs of balance and disequilibrium as metaphors for health and illness in which restoration serves as the goal of care. From older cultural traditions we learn of flows, fluids, and their disturbances as causal explanations of illness, and from physics we learn the notion of resilience to indicate the patient's capacity to recover from illness and trauma.

In Chapter 9 we shift our attention from words to their modes of transmission. Our Western cultural tradition tends to privilege talking over listening. Yet, a series of interviews with patients revealed that the most valued attribute in seeking a physician is the caregiver's capacity to listen. Listening is not simply a means to gain relevant information from a person seeking care. Careful listening indicates genuine engagement by the physician and transmits an intention to provide care. Colleagues from psychiatry and pastoral care have taught us that the acts of talking and listening are themselves means to restoration and healing.

The most remarkable instance of the power of words is that of the placebo. Regarded as interference by some pharmacologists and acts of deception by young medical students, placebos are the most impressive and least appreciated example of the impact of language in therapy. Clinicians embody the placebo effect, yet remain skeptical of its power. We try to discern the reasons for this paradox, and then review the generic presence of the placebo effect in clinical care and its putative causal mechanisms. Chapter 10 offers a comparison between drug therapies and the effects of placebos and concludes with the concept that words have the power to help or harm. We must therefore consider a framework best described as a pharmacology of words.

We briefly consider the trope of time. The common expression that time is money attests to its value as a metaphysical commodity. Time is both minutes on a watch and a perception of time invested in caring and care. Time can be understood as an enacted metaphor with unspoken yet clear meanings. We have witnessed the advent of stroboscopic medicine in which clinical care is provided in short flashes of minutes after weeks to book an appointment and hours in a waiting room. This is not unique to medicine since the societal metronome seems to have accelerated inexorably, hastened by the Web and abbreviated communiques over social media. Are these innovations a boon or burden for clinical practice, for patients and their physicians?

Part IV, Healing the Language and the Language of Healing, returns to a consideration of the patient–physician relationship in Chapter 11 and the various models that have been developed to describe this focal point of clinical care. In Chapter 12 we see how the lens of language offers a view of clinical medicine that is steeped in words and discourse and reiterates the importance of linguistic tropes to the understanding and care of persons who are ill. The book closes with the following question: If the prevalent military metaphors undermine and obstruct much-needed solutions to the current state of health care, thoroughly imbued with inappropriate language and its consequences, then how do we heal the metaphors that constitute an ailing system? Our challenge is to reframe the clinical relationship to foreground awareness, listening, reflection, and a renewed attentiveness to the power of words and their impact for good and ill in order to fulfill the mission of care.

I

LANGUAGE IN CONTEXT

1
The Lens of Language

The man arrived suffering from abdominal pain. Examination confirmed the diagnosis of acute cholecystitis—an inflamed gall bladder filled with stones. The attending surgeon scheduled the necessary simple operation for that afternoon. However, as soon as he heard the word surgery, *the patient became visibly distraught and announced his decision to leave the hospital immediately. The surgeon, puzzled by this turn of events, demanded that the patient sign a form accepting responsibility for refusing the recommended treatment. The young medical student delegated to complete the necessary documentation was able to engage the patient in a quiet discussion that uncovered the origins of his distress. Forty years earlier, the then ten-year-old patient and his mother were reassured that their father and husband required a "simple" operation—one that led to an unforeseen complication and intraoperative death.*

—Vignette from the television series *ER*

Medical care happens in the interactions between patient and physician in a virtual place called the doctor–patient relationship. The word *relationship* connotes something more than a simple act of communication and transfer of information. It harbors a sense of kinship, suffused with mutual goals, interests, and meanings. The simple, yet important, act of communication and the deeper, intersubjective clinical relationship are both made possible by language. However, these two kinds of interactions, communicative and relational, are different in structure and intention and mediated by different linguistic forms. The direct inquiry of a medical history that seeks to ascertain factual information about the patient's symptoms, their nature, duration, location, and quality, and collect demographic data such as age, occupation, domicile, and previous illnesses tends to make use of a simple descriptive linguistic form. This mode is used in science, mathematics, and logic to gather facts and describe specific details of the natural world. To provide clarity, transparent usage, and definitions that are readily shared by the community of peers, the words utilized are simple and generally denotative. This form avoids tropes whose intent may be figurative and less than immediately transparent.

The second linguistic formulation is grounded in an understanding that language is not simply designative of things as they are but can work to create new frames and ideas. As the philosopher Charles Taylor describes in his book, *The Language Animal*, language is constitutive of the world we inhabit. Words can bring into being thoughts, ideas, and formulations that could not exist before the words are articulated in a particular way. These words are often indirect and polysemous, that is, imbued with many possible meanings and uses. Such language requires interpretation and a hermeneutic stance on the part of the listener and reader. Words are linked to webs of allusions and understandings, which may require unpacking to become evident. They may be freighted with additional baggage of meanings that depend on context—both internal, that is, within the sentence or story, or external, the surroundings within which the events unfold and the story is narrated.

Take the word *triangle*. It denotes a certain geometric shape and its mathematical form and descriptive uses are clear and easily shared. By contrast, a triangle in a tale of romance and intrigue is, in human terms, a far more complex arrangement whose meaning is dependent on the participants and the contexts in which the purported events took place and in which the story is told.

The vignette that introduced this chapter serves to distinguish these two modes of language in the clinical setting. The diagnosis of cholecystitis was based on a traditional mode of taking the patient's history—that is, a series of questions designed to ascertain the relevant facts, in this instance, the duration and locus of discomfort and the factors that exacerbate the pain. A physical exam noting tenderness below the right rib cage made worse by deep inspiration confirmed the preliminary diagnosis of gall bladder inflammation and perhaps an ultrasound displayed the presence of gallstones. The interaction is couched in simple, clear questions directed to ascertain relatively straightforward information or evidence that may fulfill the diagnostic criteria for cholecystitis. The interaction between patient and physician is unimodal rather than bidirectional. While it is technically a dialogue in that two participants are involved, it is hardly a conversation. It is more akin, perhaps, to an oral examination or a spoken questionnaire. The interaction is goal directed, primarily, though not exclusively, to the objectives of the physician, and is rather pragmatic. In that sense, it appropriately uses the designative linguistic mode of the inductive scientist.

We can now contrast this mode of linguistic interaction with that of the medical student gaining an understanding of the patient's rather dramatic reaction. The aim was to decipher the specific meaning of the word *surgery* for the patient in whom it elicited a surprising response. This inquiry entailed a degree of intellectual curiosity on the part of the student and a willingness to suspend judgment, coupled with a sense of responsibility to the needs of the patient. While the word *surgery* may have seemed straightforward to the surgeon, it evidently entailed very powerfully affective meanings for the patient. Even apparently simple words are embedded in networks of allusions and meanings and carry resonances of history and usage, both societal and personal. Many such semantic linkages are shared, sometimes widely in a society and at times within specific cultural or linguistic communities. However, as in this vignette, words may have more cryptic backdrops and may be attended by idiosyncratic triggers. The simple designative function of a word does not elucidate such private and unique links. It is also evident that the power of a word is intimately linked to the context of use, both historical and current. That is, the connotations or extensions of the word *surgery* are inexorably linked for this person to a potently traumatic event. The power of this recollection stems not simply from the death of the patient's father, but rather that it took place after reassurances that the operation is a minor procedure. To unearth the private metaphor embedded in the patient's memory that simple surgery is death entailed a process of interpretation on the part of the student.

How can we best describe this clinical modality intended to gain an understanding of the thoughts of the patient? We can imagine that to initiate any productive interaction with a patient in turmoil and anxious to leave the hospital necessitates a calm and quiet space for a conversation between the participants and an unhurried time frame. The opening questions may be cautious, providing a space of silence and permitting the patient to initiate the conversation. In the scenario just described, the questions posed by the student, in contrast to the directed interrogation of the initial diagnostic process, were open-ended and intended to initiate a dialogue. The goal is to gain insight into the genesis of the patient's reaction without once again evoking a fraught response. In this instance, the interaction is a genuine bidirectional dialogue. Neither the direction of the conversation nor its outcome is clear or foreseeable at the outset. There is a need to gain as much information as possible and then extract the relevant details. Careful listening is crucial to the task, coupled with an openness to possibilities and only tentative, hesitant conclusions on the part of the listener. Opening questions may be, for example, "Please tell me how you feel," or "May we talk about what happened when you came to the hospital?" This format invites the patient to couch his or her answer as a narrative, rather than as a simple phrase or sentence. It is the first of several stories that will be required to gain the requisite understanding. Indeed, this latent web of meanings may be hidden to the patient, as well as to the clinician. It may not be evident at first that *surgery* was the evocative word, and hence attention to nuance, tone, and embodied gestures is important. The early sense that the turning point of the patient's story was not the diagnosis of cholecystitis but rather the decision to proceed to surgery afforded a growing sense of the locus of the problem. Rather than focusing the discussion, the student expanded the space around this notion of surgery and invited the patient to recall previous illnesses, visits to physicians, and other prior experiences. As the conversation continued, the patient and student could together come to understand the patient's childhood experience and how this led to a dark set of resonances to the word *surgery*. For the student, this may entail a sympathetic understanding of the patient's emotional plight and a provisional entry into the patient's world and mindset. Thus, both an affective and a cognitive apprehension of the patient's narrative are needed. To reach that stage of engagement necessitates establishing a degree of trust on the part of the patient, who, in this case, sensed the commitment of the student—or, to use a different phrase, a sense of attunement between the participants.

This careful, stepwise, and dialogic process of interpretation is the hermeneutic method, originally used to describe the exegesis and analysis of biblical and other religious texts. The scholar endeavors to grasp both the overt and allusive meanings of individual words and phrases, in the context of the overall literary work. This entails an openness to the many potential meanings of a word or phrase, its ambiguities, history of usage, and sources of accreted understandings. The dialogue in such instances is between the scholar and the layered texts. In our clinical example, the conversation is between the two participants though the objective is the same—namely, grasping the allusive and idiosyncratic meaning of the word and its context in the life history of the person. The process is painstaking and requires following a spider's web of intentions and resonances. A single strand may be tenuous, but the net is strong. It is the antithesis of a reductionist, just-the-facts stance and entails enriched and contextualized rather than stripped-away, simplistic understandings. The hermeneutic method helps us understand a traditional aphorism that the patient is a text to be read by the physician. At first glance, this may suggest a rather passive role for the patient in the clinical encounter as an open book with a clear message. However, the hermeneutic scholar engages in a dialogue with the cryptic text and poses questions in an effort to gain deeper understandings of latent messages and hidden meanings. The reader is reawakening the text by the queries and careful attention to the answers. While many of us take for granted that a painting or sculpture may require interpretation, we often forget that books are also works of art and may resist superficial understandings. This is, in certain respects, true of patients—we are all creations of the interplay between nature and nurture. Persons are the outcomes of inheritance, epigenetic modifications, life experiences, and personal histories. The patient exemplified at the beginning of the chapter is certainly a person with particular formative events and a resultant embodied and hidden text that can be made to speak through a reflective dialogue.

Hermeneutics is the method of the continental philosopher who wishes to know how life worlds are built. One of its foremost scholars, Hans-Georg Gadamer, noted that "the soul of hermeneutics consists in recognizing that perhaps the other is right."[1] That is, the reader must be capable of learning from the text, and the physician open to understanding the patient's perspective. That is best accomplished by a presumption on the part of the scholar/physician that the text/patient is correct and entails a reader/doctor who arrives with a tolerant mind. The implicit and powerful lesson is the need for a stance of humility on the part of the scholar or physician, members of two professions not normally celebrated for their modesty! Yet, without such a suppleness of mind, learning new things would be rather difficult. The antithesis of this approach is evident in diagnostic errors due to preconceived conclusions, premature closure, and the foolish epithet that the patient is a "poor historian."

It is useful to pause and reflect for a moment on the manner in which the clinical interaction is shaped by the two linguistic modes—the simple/designative and the expressive/hermeneutic.

They are not at odds, but complementary in purpose and contributions. The first is appropriate to simple situations or those that may require rapid responses and urgent action. It underpins a brief, pragmatic, physician-directed encounter that provides a solution to a straightforward problem and does not presuppose a lasting professional relationship. By contrast, puzzling or complex narratives require a deeper engagement and a more nuanced understanding. The interaction is dialogic, non-hierarchical, and characterized by a few, selected questions with more time devoted to attentive listening by the physician. The need for a modest and humble listener tends to generate a partnership, with patient and physician on the "same side of the desk," having dispensed with, at least temporarily, the ubiquitous, intrusive computer. The solution to the problem at hand tends to be arrived at jointly and collaboratively.

Most clinical undertakings are characterized by a blend of the two approaches and the transitions are often subtle, especially when guided by an experienced clinician who can choreograph a thoughtful pas-de-deux. This comparison underscores the idea that language constitutes different clinical modes and shapes the patient–doctor relationship and its outcomes. A perhaps simplistic illustration is the contrast between a multiple-choice exam and questions that require an extended essay response. The former uses clear, direct questions that invite demarcated responses from a pre-existing array of choices. The latter is framed by an invitation to reflect and expand on a theme and arrive at novel expositions and understandings. In the clinical setting, designative language is a pragmatic tool that provides a method of communication and transfer of information. By contrast, the expressive dimensions of language are not simply tools to enable interactions—words actually create the specific relationship as they are articulated by the participants. They shape and make possible certain realities and disclose the worlds of being of patient and physician. They permit an attunement of understanding between the clinician and patient, and the acts of interpretation enable the physician to gain a glimpse into the world of the patient. This notion stems from the description by the philosopher Martin Heidegger that language is the "house of being."[2] Entering into a language constitutes and provides access to the world we inhabit. Language is the point of view through which we become persons. The settled structures of language, semantics, and grammar are repositories of our history as humans and provide webs of meanings that we share with others within the linguistic community. Indeed, language is an interpersonal phenomenon and affords intersubjectivity with others. Thus, we are constituted by our biological grammar and our acquired languages. Language is a perspective on the world and provides stability by being shared with others. At the same time, different languages articulate the world variably by providing only partly congruent, or even non-overlapping, palettes of polysemous words, each with its residue of historical development. It then follows, to cite Taylor, that "different languages and cultures carry with them different such constellations of distinctions, each proposes its own order, its own way of 'housing' Being."[3] Yet, sufficient features of all languages are shared to afford general translatability and common understandings of certain essential concepts, many of them biological and embodied. Furthermore, as illustrated by our opening narrative, persons acquire idiosyncratic meanings and allusions though specific experiences; to borrow the Heideggerian metaphor, they furnish their "houses" with homemade psychic artifacts and reconfigure their beings with time and change. While there may not be any private languages, there clearly are private metaphors and cryptic meanings.

We each live in the house of our language that constitutes who we are as persons. Each house has its idiosyncratic design and its accumulated accoutrements and furnishings—some private and opaque, even to the inhabitant, while others are common and shared with others. This metaphor teaches us that the doctor, whose duty it is to create, or co-create, an effective patient–physician relationship, must deal with at least three requirements. The first is to gain the patient's trust to make possible a process of self-disclosure. This may enable the second desideratum—entry into the patient's house of being, albeit as a visitor or guest. Such access is afforded through dialogue and a painstaking attention to words, gestures, and embodied responses of the patient. It is akin to the glimpse one attains by a visit to a person's dwelling and a leisurely stroll through the private library. Third, as exemplified in our opening vignette, a careful and respectful inquiry into selected unusual "artifacts" in the house may unravel their histories and cryptic connotations. This stepwise undertaking can permit the attunement and shared perspectives that eliminate barriers between the participants such that the physician can better discern the genesis of the patient's illness and the ingredients to effective therapy.

The intent of clinical engagement is to gain a deep understanding of the world of the patient. The German word *Einfuhlung*, originally from the field of aesthetics, is defined as "identifying oneself with an object of contemplation,"[4] generally a work of art. This word has been translated as "empathy" and has led to the idea that the physician must step into the shoes of the patient. However, this understanding of the word misconstrues the clinical dynamic. It presumes that a visit to the house of being is tantamount to the arrival of a new tenant! Given our idiosyncratic natures, the admonition to step into the shoes of another is a foolish request and, moreover, impossible to effect. It is rather more helpful to seek a sensitivity and attentiveness to the patient so as to afford the physician a sense, both cognitive and affective, of the unfolding of the illness and the patient's experience thereof. In that sense, empathy does entail learning the emotional responses and stances of the ill person; however, this is an understanding that stops short of projection or identification. It requires a certain distance that ensures a clear-eyed view that yet does not aim for the cool disengagement that some have termed *detachment*. This state of tension requires the clinician to function at a variable mid-point between the two extremes of overidentification to the point of total immersion on the one hand and a cold, dispassionate demeanor on the other. The Oslerian stance of equanimity may indeed describe the requisite attentiveness to the cognitive and affective dimensions of the patient's narrative as it is not only told but actually lived. To do so necessitates an entry into the "house" of the patient and a hermeneutic curiosity for the subtexts. After all, the recounted narrative is an edited tale that hides as much as it reveals and is only the superficial face. And yet, this visit and the need to gain a sense of the emotional responses, and perhaps turmoil beneath, demand a clear-eyed stance to apprehend the idiographic dimensions of the story. A further benefit of the clinical stance of the middle distance is that it readily accommodates the requisite openness to the person who is ill and an appropriate respectfulness for the Other who seeks help. Engagement of physician with patient must leave space both for an expression of the suffering endured by the ill person and for the necessary reflection that precedes clinical understanding and therapy. Finally, a deeply immersed physician who is overtaken by the evident chaos and turmoil of witnessing illness can hardly provide the clinical presence that subtends healing. Engagement, rather than empathy, is what our chosen linguistic stance must create.

A Moment of Learning

An interesting comment from Gadamer helps us appreciate the impact of the interpretive process on the young student in our story. The philosopher explains, "That true experience is that which surprises us, which knocks us back, which confounds our expectations. This experience leads us to revise our expectations and opens new horizons to us."[5] It is likely that the student will long remember the conversation with the troubled patient and will have gained new allusions that will contribute to and inflect future clinical encounters. After all, the gathering of novel meanings for old words, an acquaintance with new ones, and the extension of allusive linguistic webs and metaphors constitute lifelong learning and enrich clinical experience. To be sure, coming to the clinical encounter with an open mind is not tantamount to a tabula rasa. Quite the contrary. Learning is made possible by antecedent concepts and frames that provide the Velcro to capture and incorporate new experiences and create novel thoughts. What is essential is a richness of experience coupled with an authentic openness to other persons and creative understandings. Parenthetically, this provides an important corollary for medical educators—namely, that effective clinical learning takes place in the daily encounters with a great variety of patients and their individuality, both personal and clinical.

Clinical Work

The construct of two types of linguistic frames permits us to distinguish two modalities of clinical work. The nonfigurative language that seeks to ascertain specific facts in a rapid pragmatic fashion is akin to the purposeful questions posed by an immigration agent at a border crossing. This mode has its place, though it presumes a rather straightforward, perhaps routine, clinical encounter. Yet, it has several significant limitations, perhaps even risks. What appears at first glance simple may be deceptively complex. Our clinical example is a useful illustration. Second, while an initial assessment may sometimes be routine, a therapeutic approach to resolving the problem often requires a more customized plan and hence a deeper knowledge of the patient's circumstances and contexts. Moreover, the direct stance tends to isolate a given issue and abstract it from the patient—for example, treating the gall bladder and not the person who comes for help. The expressive, dialogic linguistic mode underwrites a richer and more effective clinical encounter and is better suited to a relationship that achieves the goals of what many have termed *patient-centered medicine*. The partnership and shared responsibility avoids the question of who is in charge, not by making the parties equivalent but rather by understanding the differing, yet necessary, contributions of patient and physician. Thus, most clinical interactions are better served by the engagement between patient and physician that is created by the more nuanced, figurative, narrative mode of expressive linguistic tropes. Yet, paradoxically, as noted in the Introduction, while patients express a need for an interactive, attentive clinician, a series of contextual stresses and pressures threaten the viability of such a relational mode.

Contemporary Pressures and Threats

The engaged clinical encounter that patients seek and that physicians are duty-bound to provide is constituted by the expressive, figurative linguistic mode and requires both a particular mindset on the part of clinicians and a series of necessary, permissive contexts. The attitudes of doctors and their habits are shaped by education, experience, and the general societal milieu. Each of these three formative incubators has been increasingly beset by pressures and stresses that tend to shift clinical modes of thinking and doing toward the pragmatic, descriptive linguistic mode that mitigates against the fully engaged clinical encounter. Let us examine each in turn.

Two major methodological changes have characterized medical pedagogy over the recent past. The earlier was the widespread introduction of the problem-based curriculum that replaced traditional magisterial courses in the disciplines relevant to medicine, with content organized into discrete clinical problems to be analyzed and solved in a small-group teaching setting. The major benefit was the shift from passive, lecture-based learning to an active, participatory, curious student interacting with peers to re-enact the process of discovery of solutions to common clinical conditions. However, the learning process underwrote a positivistic, deductive approach that concurrently shifted attention to the disease or pathological process and undermined a holistic gaze toward the patient. Its pragmatic frame rewarded correct answers and a descriptive, focused attitude. A more recent development helpfully moves the focus from the content to the learner and is titled competency-based medical education (CBME). First introduced in postgraduate medical training, this innovation is now gaining attention from educators designing medical school curricula. While the problem-based method disarticulated curricular content into modules and segments, CBME dissects the anticipated knowledge and skills of learners into units and separate activities that are assessed independently. While the focus of the first is on content and the second on the learners, each is necessarily reductionist and non-holistic, and neither directs attention to the patient who seeks help. More relevant to our analysis, each tends to utilize the descriptive, analytic linguistic mode rather than the interpretive, expressive modality.

Experience in the hospital and clinic and the opportunity to meet and learn from a great and diverse array of patients is the crucible for medical education. Trainees must be afforded the setting and time in which to open a dialogue with patients, gain an understanding of their personhood, and reflect on the nature of their illnesses. They must also have sufficient opportunities to witness the course of illness over time and see firsthand the outcomes of various interventions. Yet, the modern teaching hospital is increasingly a place of short-term admissions and indeed is gauged and rewarded for ever-shorter lengths of stay. The majority of inpatients suffer from acute illnesses and are often in intensive care or postoperative situations following rapid interventions and thus not easily amenable to an afternoon's visit with a medical student. Most medical interactions with such patients are geared toward solving the problems of the day and often provided by "hospitalists" or "nocturnalists" who themselves do not provide extended care and hence are not suitable role models for continuity of care. The outpatient environment is hardly much more conducive to learning, given clinics with large waiting rooms full of persons seeking care and clinical interactions occupying time frames of a few minutes. Such medical visits are constrained to attend to one or a very few isolated problems and too often with doctors whom patients may see only once. In short, societal contexts push the majority of medical care toward the pragmatic, problem-solving discourse of the urgent care center. Certainly, such ancillary resources are fine if they are adjuncts to continuing attention by primary care providers. However, the modalities of rapid visits and acute interventions have increasingly become substitutes, rather than support mechanisms, for a longitudinal clinical engagement.

Societal trends, viewed either broadly or within the health care environment, intersect with language to influence the clinical relationship. For example, the electronic health record facilitates the accessibility of information about patients and provides a comprehensive view of encounters and test results. At the same time, the usual electronic format constrains the freedom afforded by traditional charts by encouraging telegraphic notes and making it difficult to record the clinical story with citations of the patient's own words. In addition, the acronyms and mnemonics of medical jargon complicate the transparency of the electronic record despite offering easier access—a frequent request by advocates of patient-centered medicine. A more insidious feature of computer-assisted medicine are the check-box selections and drop-down menus that are replacing free text entries by caregivers. Point- and check-boxes permit recording of elements such as duration of concerns and gravity of symptoms. However, in order to standardize for efficiency and administrative data collection, they also supplant careful clinical descriptions that attend to idiosyncratic particularities. Drop-down menus prompt physicians with lists of blood tests and other investigations in response to isolated features of a patient's presenting symptoms. Thus, the recording of the word *headache* may trigger a list of CAT scans and ancillary investigations that are stand-ins for the thoughtful clinical attention and analysis needed to comprehend the patient's story of migraine headaches. The computer encourages and perhaps even demands the descriptive pragmatic linguistic mode with its attendant simplifications and dilutions of the record. Two corollaries then follow. First, the electronic health record undermines the co-construction of a coherent narrative of illness by fragmenting the array of data into pigeonholes and boxes and by obscuring the timelines necessary to narrative understanding. Second, the constraints on free text inscriptions make it difficult for a caregiver to record the process of reasoning and interpretive steps that led to the diagnosis and treatment plans. This makes it very difficult for a consulting colleague clinician to reconstruct the prior understanding and nigh-on impossible to share such relevant insights with other members of the health care team. In effect, the narrative of illness is nowhere recorded and becomes an ephemeral object.

The development and utility of evidence-based medicine (EBM) is another instructive example of a two-edged sword with unintended consequences, viewed through our comparative lens of the two linguistic modalities. EBM is a valuable, ongoing compilation of the available empirical evidence in support of various diagnostic and therapeutic modalities and interventions. It uses the analytic and statistical tools of the epidemiologist and clinical scientist to evaluate, distill, and present the best evidence gleaned from the biomedical literature to the benefit of those developing guidelines for practice and for the physician who needs high-quality information to make decisions with and for an individual patient. Such validated data sets can improve decision-making by providing broad empirical information that a single practitioner could not reasonably gather and assess single-handedly. However, implicit in the use of EBM is a two-step process, each phase best viewed by each of the two linguistic modes. The acquisition of empirical information that forms the basis of EBM makes use of the inductive, descriptive, and pragmatic mode of clinical science. It prizes comparability, standardization, and transparent validation of the quality and utility of various clinical trials and experiments. These are crucial to the usefulness of such evidence and the assignments of levels of confidence and quality, often termed and categorized as levels of evidence, designed to assist the decision-maker. Such data sets and evaluations must necessarily represent populations, cohorts, and large treatment groups that aggregate, average, and reshape myriads of individual experiences. Therefore, the actual value in the use of guidelines and data sets is in the painstaking selection of those elements most relevant to the specific person who is the patient receiving attention.

A data set comprises a distribution of many individual data points from which overall features such as practice guidelines are abstracted and computed. By contrast, a given patient represents one of the many individual data points used to calculate the statistical conclusions. This epistemological move from the abstractions of the full data set to their application to the individual patient requires a (hermeneutic) interpretation of the constituent data sets, the resultant practice guidelines, and patient in question. Only a careful understanding of how they intersect—the aggregate data and the singular person—permits the clinician to arrive at a provisionally correct choice and recommendation. However, all too often, it is quick and expedient to simply apply the available guidelines with the assumption that since they are validated in the aggregate, they also of necessity apply to the individual patient in the specific instance. The elimination of the second, interpretive step is yet another casualty to the current hegemony of positivistic and scientistic stances that squelch narrative and interpretive understandings.

A final significant change in our societal context is that of time. The measurement and precision of time is a technical and scientific achievement that makes us believe that it is an absolute and fixed quantity. Yet, the experience of time and its phenomenological understanding are rather relative and abstract. The pace of postmodern life has accelerated and our social metronomes are ticking more quickly with each passing year. This has had a deleterious effect on our habits of language use and a consequent dilution of the strength and value of the clinical relationship. The impact of such change is evident in the continuing pleas from patients for caregivers who make a window in space–time to attend and listen. The resultant degradation of clinical presence is, of course, made worse by the accompanying shift to the descriptive language of brief questions and quicker answers and a health care system that has come to prize high volumes and short lengths of stay.

Registers and Footings

Registers refer to diverse repertoires of language that are used in interpersonal interactions. Rather than single words, registers include syntax, grammar, choice of words and phrases, tone, and degrees of formality or lack thereof. Such repertoires mark social interactions, help define hierarchies, and indicate identities of class and occupation and are thus deeply bound to social and cultural practices. Registers demarcate social strata and signal membership in groups and professional orders, and both reflect and structure interpersonal relationships. They may create boundaries between different groups—for example, physicians and patients—and impair communication and sharing of understandings. However, a sensitivity and attention to the differences in registers can work to transcend such barriers and forge necessary alliances, both social and professional.

While registers refer to the nature of the discourse between or among individuals, *footing* is a figurative word that describes the nature of their social and interpersonal relationships. Such footings may be hierarchical, egalitarian, intimate, familiar, professional, comradely, hostile, deferential, detached, and transactional, to name only a few. Registers and footings are not fixed and can vary even for the same two persons, depending on situation and context. For example, father and son can be on an authoritarian footing and use a carefully chosen register when discussing academic records, and an egalitarian footing and an informal, buddy register when fishing together. By contrast, the father is not likely to use his professional register of legal language at home or regard his daughter as a client.

Our interest in registers and footings lies in the notion that both are enacted in language, both verbal and nonverbal, and both shape and constitute the clinical (and other) relationships that are at the heart of medicine. One excellent example is the characteristics of the various narratives that are related by patients and doctors. The story of illness a person shares with her neighbor, the one she records in her diary, and the one told to the physician all stem from similar symptoms and concerns, yet the registers in which they are couched vary considerably. In turn, the narrative of the physician explaining to the patient her understanding and significance of the illness, the text in the case record, the entry to the electronic health file, and the story told to the colleague consultant over lunch are all in different registers. In each set of instances, the chosen discourse reflects the intent of the interaction, the relative footings of the interlocutors, and the social norms that govern such relationships. While these may seem complex, the selection of register is often one of learned habits and the result of long experience with the cultural norms of a given social community. However, linguistic registers and the footings that they enable and mark require reflective attention and thoughtful choices by physicians and other caregivers.

Physicians are often criticized for a paternalistic and authoritarian stance toward patients. And indeed, that may at times be the case. At the other end of the spectrum, some patients and their physicians prefer a more informal, colloquial, and first name–based relationship that is more generally the norm among old friends and families. This contrast helps us notice that there is no single and simple answer for all and, as is often the case, the optimal register is specific to the person, with antecedent histories and personal metrics of social ease.

This spectrum of possibilities, rather than black-and-white choices, helps us identify an array of registers along several axes that are relevant to the clinical setting. Before examining several of these, we should recall our guiding principles gleaned from the analysis of linguistic modes. First, clinical practice must abide by the norms of bespoke tailoring rather than off-the-rack clothing—we craft a custom-designed garment that suits the persona and needs of the individual patient. Second, the craftsman must take the measure of the man (or woman)—the tailor or couturier using a tape measure and the physician using the skills of listening and assessment. Only by careful attention can the physician discern the character of the person seeking care and thereby attend to the appropriate stances and registers. Last, the client has the prerogative to choose the fabric and style, yet the physician has the duty to guide these choices and ensure that they are the best options for the patient.

While a respectful attitude of attention is a sine qua non in all clinical encounters, other aspects must be calibrated in a partnership, for which the clinician assumes prime responsibility. Each selection along an axis is effectively characterized by a specific register and also engenders an associated footing. For example, some patients prefer a physician who serves as a friendly provider of expertise, advice, and information and permits the patient to make choices and important decisions. Some have described this as patient-guided care, as the next stage beyond patient-centered medicine. By contrast, many patients find security in a physician who is more directive in decision-making and seek comfort in accepting a more authoritative and perhaps, paternalistic clinician. No doubt, such divergences depend on the patient's habits in dealing with the world, prior experiences with illness and health care, and the nature and quality of an antecedent relationship with the physician. Such factors also inflect the spectrum between a formal, somewhat reserved clinical persona and one who is more friendly, informal, and readily accessible by email in a rather familiar fashion. For some, these choices may depend on the nature of the illness, with the former footing preferred for single consultations for serious conditions and the latter for ongoing low-intensity care. As noted previously, registers may include nonverbal messages and semiotic tropes. Some pediatricians opt for informal garb in the hospital and clinic and avoid white coats and business attire that may appear strange to children. Other clinicians insist that dress-down Fridays do not belong in a serious health care setting and note that a clean and starched white coat sends a signal of professionalism and competence. There are also findings in the psychology literature that wearing a white coat, that is, "donning the habit," instills a sense of self-esteem in a young physician so attired.

A frequent question from medical students who are taught to be attentive to boundaries in clinical situations is how they can express their genuine concern for their patients while maintaining the appropriate clinical distance. How can they address the tension that characterizes the dilemmas of a requisite detachment versus the necessary clinical engagement? Again, the answer lies in a customized stance that takes into account the patient's specific needs, age, and wishes. Between the ends of this axis whose poles are breaching personal boundaries, some of them inviolable even with consent, and a robotic demeanor at the other extreme, is a long continuum with nuanced and varying options. Another metric for the tension is the physician's risk of emotional immersion that may incapacitate an ability to provide care and the need to serve as a barometer to the patient's emotional state as an index to diagnosis and management. Once again, a reflective analysis of the needs of the person who is ill and the duty of the physician to address those needs will serve as guides to a careful calibration of the registers and footings that shape the clinical relationship and the linguistic choices that do the work.

2
From Words to "Making Up People"

When asked to bring an artifact to class to illustrate an interest in the language of medicine, one student brought a small hand mirror to class. The mirror, she explained, is what she uses to reflect on her questions: "How do my patients see me? What do they see when I am with them?"

—McGill medical student

Our interest in words and language stems from their influence on the clinical interaction between patient and doctor. More generally, we seek to understand how language both reflects and shapes societal and cultural attitudes and stances in health care. Our task now is to delve into specific instances of linguistic potency.

Responsibility and Blame

Humans prefer to know how and why things happen and seek clear explanations of causality. We choose to attribute events to simple factors, try to avoid ambiguity, and are made uncomfortable by the unexpected. One of the interesting challenges in medical education is to integrate the robust clarity of scientific explanations for physiological phenomena with the complexity and uncertainty of clinical care for individual patients. A corollary of our quest for linear causal connections is a desire to assign responsibility when things go awry. This need is so powerful that cause-and-effect links are often accepted as true despite overwhelming evidence to the contrary. A sad example is the decline in childhood vaccinations because of a mistaken belief that such vaccines account for the increasing prevalence of autism. We are disconcerted by the uncertain etiology of this developmental illness and seek an explanation. Many well-meaning parents are unhappy with the difficulties in dealing with and gaining access to health care. Their mistrust in the sometimes chaotic system of care, coupled with fear of a mysterious ailment, leads to dire consequences for all children, both vaccinated and not. The resultant recrudescence of measles is not a failure of medicine as science but a catastrophe of societal attitudes and misplaced blame. It is also a failure of adequate communication between the profession and those whom we serve, individually and collectively. Other significant examples of inappropriate interventions due to lapses in joint understanding abound. Antibiotic prescriptions for viral illnesses and unnecessary Caesarean sections for healthy pregnant women are often the result of a misguided alliance between caregivers and patients.

Attention to words and spoken language in the clinical setting reveals something more insidious—a shift of responsibility and blame by caregivers onto unwitting, quite innocent, patients. Experiments have revealed that medical students are unable to comply with detailed prescriptions to consume a variety of pills three or four times a day, despite straightforward instructions. Not surprising then that elderly patients may unintentionally omit some medications over the course of a month or more. And yet, when patients have not taken all their medications as prescribed, they are described as "non-compliant," suggesting an intentional breach of instructions and hinting at a less than diligent desire to get better. Another instance comes from an anagram of compliant, namely, complaint. The phrase "chief complaint" has long served in medical charts to label the patient's reason for seeking care. This, of course, implicitly compares a person who comes to a clinic in need of medical attention with an unhappy customer returning a purchase to a department store. To counter this derogatory connotation, some medical educators have recommended the use of "chief concern" as a more suitable and respectful descriptor.

There is another class of usage that ascribes agency to patients to explain unfortunate circumstances and complications. "The patient is a poor historian" is a comment used by a resident or student to excuse a less than coherent clinical story. It may well be true that an ill, confused patient is unable to supply all the medically relevant details in a clear narrative. However, this ignores the possibility that the young physician is less than adept at eliciting such information and co-constructing and presenting a cogent history of the illness. More overt examples of attributed responsibility are instructive. A blood clot that arises in the deep veins of the legs and travels in the bloodstream to the lungs—a pulmonary embolus—is a common complication in a bedridden patient and may cause an acute and life-threatening event. Another emergency situation is a sudden decline in blood pressure in a sick person. At early morning wards rounds the question, "Did anything happen last night?" may be greeted with the following: "Bed 3 threw an embolus and bed 6 dropped her blood pressure!" Leaving aside for the moment the replacement of the human by a number, such informal descriptions are rarely noted in the written record but are elements of a medical vernacular dialect common in hospital wards and clinics. They attribute direct agency to the patient and thereby assign blame for the unfortunate complication. They also shift attention away from the physicians and other caregivers whose actions or omissions may have precipitated the sequence of events.

A more insidious assignment of responsibility is the result of well-intentioned efforts to promulgate the early detection of breast and other cancers. In the 1950s major public campaigns for cancer detection and prevention were based on a premise that early interventions were essential for good outcomes. Advertising by cancer societies urged attention to what were considered early warning signs with admonitions to search for any change in a wart or mole. Public awareness campaigns were directed primarily to women who were encouraged to seek annual pap smears, regular mammography, and breast self-examinations. These efforts at early detection of malignancies in response to what seemed to be rising risks were directed at patients, or more accurately, healthy persons with cryptic, or preclinical disease. The net effect was to assign responsibility to healthy persons for ensuring that these screening procedures were carried out in a timely fashion and on a recurrent basis. Some may have been pleased with the notion of taking responsibility for their own health. Others, by contrast, may have suffered the added insult of self-blame when a lesion was detected after a longer than recommended period between screening visits. Rather than developing a means of shared engagement and accountability, these well-meaning efforts shifted the responsibility to patients and healthy persons. At the same time, the 1950s and 1960s still supported a rather hierarchical medicine in which doctors made decisions and patients were relegated to a more passive role. This exacerbated the tension between accepting active responsibility for mitigating risk and passively accepting major interventions, for example, radical mastectomies—all the while leaving the fearful, newly diagnosed woman to worry whether her breast self-examination had been inadequate or belated.

It is reasonable to consider that personal responsibility for health is a boon, not a burden. However, a shared management of risks mitigates a sense of guilt and blame when things go awry. After all, that seems to be the norm in other professional relationships. Teachers, accountants, and lawyers assume a measure of responsibility in dealing with matters that can affect our welfare. In medicine, attributions of risks seem to require legal processes of malpractice claims. Why does our language reflect the shift of responsibility to patients in the medical arena? Perhaps the consequences in medicine are more serious and, potentially, life-threatening, thus evincing a more defensive and self-protective stance by caregivers. Or, the words we have described may reflect a distancing from the suffering that shapes the perceptions of clinicians. Whatever the reasons, an attention to the language we use is mandatory if we are to avoid its ill effects on the lives of patients and their capacities to cope with illness.

Reciprocity

When physicians provide care for patients, they often misconstrue the exchange as unidirectional in focus and attention. Patients describe their concerns and needs, and doctors provide advice, prescriptions, and management. Physicians are aware of the need to assess their patients to ascertain their states of health but forget that they themselves are also being keenly observed and measured. Do they ask themselves whether their demeanor, dress, and clinic surroundings transmit a sense of assurance and confidence? Does their body language signal that things are proceeding well, or does their vocal intonation suggest a reason to worry? Patients and their families are in a heightened state of awareness and concern, especially after a sudden onset of illness. They seek clues and signs from their caregivers that may indicate the gravity of the situation, and they try to read the skills and experience of their physicians in the behaviors they observe. The student who realized that asking an evidently homeless person what he does for a living may in fact be perceived as a criticism, rather than a request for information, was led to reflect on how she and her fellow young clinicians are seen by those for whom they provide care, hence the mirror in our opening anecdote. Does their language, both verbal and embodied, express detachment or engagement, a hierarchical perspective or an egalitarian stance, a view from above or the eye contact of someone sharing a common perspective? Clinicians learn to be observant and take note of the patient's habitus and gait, of the pale skin of anemia and the flaccid muscles of malnutrition. This intensely directed attention is necessary for best clinical practice—perhaps it also blunts the physician's sensibility and regard to the reciprocal gaze of the patient seeking care. Or, the lack of attention to the presentation of the self may be a result of pragmatic detachment and a need for short visits and focused care. The paradox is that becoming adept at reading the signs and signals emanating from patients does not automatically translate into a parallel awareness of self. Acuity of clinical perception need not be, but often is, accompanied by a deafness of the caregiver to the messages evident to the patient. Thus, three kinds of reflective attention to language are incumbent on the physician in the clinical setting. First, of course, is careful listening to the words and thoughts of the patient in order to comprehend the story of the illness and its meaning for the person. Second is the careful choice of the words directed to the patient and family with an ear for the effect of spoken utterances on their understanding of the process of the illness and its effect on their lives. Third is the concern raised by the student's story—a reflective concern with the impact of the physician's demeanor and embodied expressions eagerly and anxiously deciphered by the patient.

Infantilizing Language

The effect of the performative dimension of language and the impact of intonation and attitude of the speaker on the listener are clearly evident in living facilities for the elderly with dementias. Such elderly persons sometimes respond with aggressive behaviors, such as kicking, biting, and screaming, when nurses attempt to provide care, such as feeding, dressing and moving from bed to chair. Observers noticed that these difficult behaviors occurred far more often when the attendants used infantilizing language when dealing with the elderly patients.[1] Words, phrases, and intonation usually reserved for dealing with infants and small children, such as "There, there, how are we today?" or "Have we had our breakfast this morning?" or "Wakey, wakey, time to get up," were more likely to elicit aggressive behavioral responses compared with neutral language or quiet requests. As far as we can tell, these elderly patients with dementia did not grasp the literal meaning of the words of the nurses who provided care. Rather, they may have sensed the unintentionally pejorative tones of the infantile words and the resultant degradation of dignity and respect. Even when the cognitive capacity to interpret semantic meanings is impaired, the affective dimensions of prosody and tone are still registered and evoke behavioral responses. Patients may comprehend far more than we imagine, even when comatose or living with impaired cognition.

Small Words and Big Impact

Patients often visit physicians' offices with more than one concern in mind. They may seek advice on several issues and generally present only one of these in response to the opening question of the interview. As a result, important health care worries may not be addressed in the absence of follow-up probes later in the discussion. If a patient is prompted by being asked, "Is there is *some*thing else you wish to review during the visit?" then the majority of previously noted concerns are revealed. However, the question, "Is there *any*thing else you wish to review during the visit?" is relatively ineffective in eliciting such concerns. The two formats, *some*thing and *any*thing, are often used interchangeably in medical interviews, though the difference between them in eliciting significant health care concerns is quite surprising.[2] The explanation offered by linguists is that the prefix *some-* tends to elicit a "yes," while *any-* is generally part of negatively framed sentences and elicits a "no" response. The latter is described as having negative polarity. This difference is clinically relevant in that the added concerns are often non-trivial and warrant medical attention. Experts who construct survey questionnaires are aware of the power of small words and the impact of syntax in shaping responses. Such linguistic elements are no less important in the daily life of the clinic.

Framing

The power of small words is one example of a more general phenomenon of framing, well-studied in the field of psychology and often referred to as cognitive bias. Framing describes the effect of language in shaping or guiding our perception and understanding of things. As we shall see, this is part of the rhetorical power of metaphors. However, simple, non-metaphoric labels and seemingly neutral terms can have a similar effect. A research questionnaire presented patients with a description of a person with a run-of-the-mill acute respiratory illness.[3] Three different diagnostic labels were assigned to the same clinical description in three test groups: chest cold, viral upper respiratory infection, or bronchitis. The group reading a scenario culminating in a diagnosis of bronchitis were twice as likely to indicate the need for a prescription for an antibiotic compared with the other two diagnoses. Quite simply, a patient's request for an unnecessary antibiotic is directly influenced by the physician's choice among equivalent diagnostic terms. Thus, attentiveness to language by physicians may contribute to a diminution of the overuse of antibiotics for children and adults and thereby reduce the burgeoning prevalence of multiply-resistant bacterial strains.

Several unanticipated findings emerged from a qualitative study of interviews with women whose tumors were tested for gene expression in an attempt to tailor the choice of chemotherapy for breast cancer in a clinical trial.[4] First, the investigators used the terms *genetic* and *genomic* interchangeably, while some subjects presumed the latter term was synonymous with hereditary. This sparked concerns of the genetic transmission of cancer from mother to daughters. Second, not all tumor samples could be successfully analyzed. In some instances, the lab result of "not done" or "not interpretable" was misunderstood by the patient as indicating an extremely negative prognosis and the subsequent ineligibility for the clinical trial left the woman feeling abandoned. These are clearly serious consequences for the welfare of these women who are confronted with unintended distress caused by word choice in addition to the demands of coping with serious illness. Once again, such ill effects are unintended by clinicians and researchers and constitute a type of corollary or bystander damage from potent, or perhaps, toxic language.

Just A Medical Student, or JAMS

Part of the informal lore among medical students is the acronym, JAMS, or Just a Medical Student. This is a self-deprecating phrase students use to remind themselves of their lowly place in the pecking order of the caregiver team in a hospital or clinic. It may be tinged with some bitterness when a student's contribution to a team discussion is neither solicited nor appreciated when provided. In this setting, the concept may reflect the silencing of the student's voice by an authoritarian supervisor who represents a less than ideal role model and mentor.

The word *just* is evident when a medical student declares, "There was nothing I could do, so I just sat and talked with the patient." Or, "I just let her cry." This single word speaks volumes when expressed by students in a clinical setting. It underscores the tacit lesson that technical acts such as prescribing medications constitute doing something but spending time with a patient, talking and listening, is distinct from actual medical care. The students' own inclinations are often to spend more time with their patients—after all, this is what attracted them to a career in medicine. However, students working on a busy ward are often instructed to avoid spending too much time with patients, as there is real work to be done. This is the first of several paradoxes students may witness—that talking with patients is not medicine. Students appreciate that they are considered to have more free time than overworked residents and busy attending staff physicians, leading to a paradoxical conclusion: the more important you are, the less time you spend with patients, and those with power have little time. This underscores an antithetical role model who minimizes contact with patients and concurrently undermines what students are taught in the classroom. Theoretical course offerings on doctoring and clinical skills celebrate relational knowledge and skills. By contrast, students who attempt to implement such lessons in the clinical setting may, surprisingly, elicit criticism from mentors and seniors. Thus, students can experience cognitive dissonance and tensions among what they are taught, their own burgeoning identities as physicians, and what they sometimes witness in training. As the scholar Anna Romer observed in her study of senior medical students, they come to learn that they will not "be rewarded for the time and energy they invest when engaged in moments of healing."[5] As one student noted of his clinical experience in the hospital, "you can get away with being brusque ... you can't get away with bad medicine."[6] Patients are in a heightened state of awareness and attuned to the choice of words they hear; they listen intently for meanings that concern their health and welfare. Similarly, students in training are in a liminal state—they are excited to finally have the opportunity to interact directly with patients and concurrently vulnerable to the critiques they perceive regarding their own behaviors. All the more when they are taken to task for following the norms they were taught in the classroom. Thus, an analysis of the simple word *just* as articulated by medical students in training uncovers an important mindset of contemporary clinical pedagogical experience that warrants the serious attention of medical educators.

Linguistic Relativity

Language constitutes and shapes the world in which we live. It is then plausible that different languages engender disparate experiences and may not only shape perception but also lead to different thoughts. The notion that language shapes thought, rather than simply reflecting our thinking, is attributed to Benjamin Whorf and Edward Sapir, who formulated this hypothesis between the 1930s and the 1950s. It is rooted in work in transcultural anthropology, more particularly, in observed differences between peoples of the European-Western world and indigenous peoples of developing countries who were the subjects of study of anthropologists in the mid-twentieth century. In its early formulations, the Whorf-Sapir hypothesis predicted that how individuals perceive colors would depend on the words used in their language to identify colors and the gradations among them. In other words, purple can be seen only by persons whose language contains a word for that color. Empirical tests by psychologists over many decades failed to show major differences in how persons see colors despite diverse semantic labels. Nonetheless, there are subtle differences that demonstrate the validity of the hypothesis in an attenuated, weak form, but not in its original strong prediction that language shapes all thinking.

While such effects were difficult to show empirically for references to objective observations of the natural world, linguistic differences are readily demonstrable for abstract thought and culturally laden phenomena. The term *linguistic relativity*[7] has been applied to such interactions between words and the perceptions of objects to which they refer. A common example are gendered nouns, especially those for inanimate objects, that have grammatical genders in some languages and whose linguistic assignments are independent of the properties of the objects they denote. For example, German considers a bridge to be a feminine noun, while Spanish classes it as masculine. In keeping with these arbitrary grammatical assignments, German speakers describe a bridge as elegant and fragile, while native Spanish speakers choose strong and towering to describe the same object. Another instance are the poetic connotations of the color white for English speakers for whom it suggests purity, brides, and weddings, while for native speakers of Mandarin, white invites thoughts of mortality and death. Conversely, red in Chinese is the color of celebrations, while in English it evokes pictures of trauma, both physical and moral. Such linguistic effects are well known to those who produce and sell pharmaceutical products and choose light blue and other muted pastel colors for sedatives and bright red and green hues for antidepressants.

It is not surprising that the phenomenon of linguistic relativity and the subtle influences of words on perception and experience are less often associated with the descriptive, concrete language used in the natural sciences. Yet, even in this domain one can discern frameworks that shift and reshape views of the world. Thomas Kuhn argued that shared views of the natural world are possible only within a given paradigm. The advent of a new formulation opens a vista to a different world. In fact, it is near impossible to see beyond an engrained paradigm—it takes a genius with a novel conceptual insight expressed in language to create a new framework for understanding and, with it, a new world.

If the strong form of the Whorf-Sapir hypothesis that language is deterministic of thought is a variant that finds little contemporary support, the weaker form that language shapes and molds thought finds special resonance in the domain of figurative and abstract words and thoughts. After all, the constitutive capacity of language creates the world we perceive and understand. Hence, different cultures constitute and express themselves through language that generates the diverse worlds described in the work of cultural anthropologists.

The important instances of linguistic relativity in medicine are found in the different modalities of language among what can be described as micro-cultures within a single, though not homogeneous, linguistic group. Let us begin with the simplest division of groups or micro-cultures—those who are well, those who are ill, and physicians with a duty to provide care. Each group has its own lexicon, registers, and metaphors, though all share a common language, let us say, English. The particular variety of a language used by a given social group or category, that is, its lexicon, syntax, and even rhetorical and prosodic character, are its *sociolect*—the dialect, or way of speaking of that group. We have previously described the differences in registers among groups and how these influence social communication and capacity for mutual understandings. Registers also affect how persons see each other in interactions and talk. Indeed, the student who brought the mirror to class wondered how the patient sees her, given her habitus, demeanor, and communicative register. Hence, differences in sociolect may impede communication between individuals from different micro-cultures.

These sociolinguistic barriers presume only that diverse lexicons describe a common world in different fashions and hence would be the case even if language simply reflected different modes of thinking and perceiving the same world. However, the Whorf-Sapir hypothesis, even in its weak formulation, teaches us that language and sociolects shape thoughts and thereby constitute varieties of worlds. Communication is not a simple matter of translation across or between sociolects; it is, rather, a challenge of interpretation and hermeneutic understanding in order to glimpse the world of the other and thereby grasp some sense of how it may be to live in that world. This deepens the challenge of social communication in general and underscores a special requirement for sharing words and thoughts in the clinical setting. In ordinary descriptive talk, the interlocutors generally share a common view of the world and can agree, for example, that there are four books on the table with no need for interpretation. By contrast, when a patient describes a symptom, say, a headache, to a physician, only the superficial information is readily shared and rooted in a common view. For example, the question, "How many days have you had the pain?" may receive a straightforward, numerical response. By contrast, to respond to "How much does it hurt?" requires words familiar to both speakers, yet with different semantic resonances for each. The word *acute* when referring to recent onset is easy to share; when pointing to severity, shared understanding is rather more difficult. Nonetheless, by using numerical scales and comparators, assessment of pain becomes possible. However, when the question becomes "What does this mean?" translation becomes impossible, though interpretation may find traction. We must first accept that for the patient, the word *pain* may conjure up a world of an interrupted life and fear of a brain tumor. For the physician, the same word presents a quotidian diagnostic conundrum that is part of daily life, not an ominous intrusion. This divide may be inadvertently widened when the surgeon recommends a simple biopsy. Many a patient has pointed out that operations are simple for surgeons but never trivial for patients. We may recall the story of the previous chapter and its special resonances of the word *surgery* for the patient with a particular history and personal memory. In that instance, the word connoted an operative disaster. This also points to the existence of *idiolects*, namely, a linguistic system of one person, differing in some important way from that of all others of the same sociolect. The challenge of idiosyncratic, private meanings and cryptic metaphors necessitates both the recognition of linguistically shaped individual worlds and the clinical obligation for hermeneutic acts of interpretation. Virginia Woolf captured the linguistic challenges with, "let a sufferer try to describe a pain in his head to a doctor and language at once runs dry."[8] Clinical work entails entry into the lifeworld of the patient through thoughtful engagement with the text of the narrative embedded in the being of the person—in other words, close reading of the text that is the patient.

A framework that may help us understand this act of interpretation that mediates between diverse worlds is that of semiosis that involves the cooperation of three elements: a sign, its object, and its interpretant. In clinical medicine, the sign is a subjective report by the patient (symptom) or objective trace (sign) of illness. The interpretant is the concept generated by the sign in the mind of the interpreter, for example, the physician, with respect to the object. In this instance, the object may be the illness or (preferably) the person who is ill. Interpretation is the interaction among the three elements to elicit a richer meaning in the mind of the interpreter. This is akin to traditional textual hermeneutics in which the reader is the interpreter, the words on the page are the sign, and the object is the embedded meaning or the work as whole. To take a concrete example, consider the appearance of a yellow tinge to the skin or the whites of the eyes, known as jaundice. The most overt reading of the sign is an obstruction to the flow of bile resulting in a yellowed appearance. For the physician, the sign evokes a chain of reasoning to reach a causal understanding of the illness within. It is reasonable to presume that this sign resonates somewhat differently for each interpreter. Each physician will see the situation somewhat differently, depending on prior experience with patients with jaundice, the institution within which the interaction takes place, and the prevalence of certain illnesses in the contextual community. All these contingent factors indicate that the sign, jaundice, evokes different images in the mind of each physician, whose mental map is the result of an aggregation of allusions of the word and its particular connotations. Moreover, how jaundice is understood is inflected by how the particular patient appears to the interpreting physician. A person whose dress and demeanor may be suggestive of homelessness may trigger a pejorative reaction toward a presumed drug addict or alcoholic. Of course, all such initial images will then shape the course and nature of the questions addressed to the patient in order to decipher the nature of the cause.

We must consider other possible constellations of the triad of sign, object, and interpretant in the mind of the interpreter. This framing can also showcase the concerns of the patient as interpreter attempting to decipher the signs on the physician's face to get a sense of the implications of jaundice for the patient's own future. This is, of course, a more difficult hermeneutic act, given physicians' common demeanor of dispassionate detachment and a tendency to conceal concerns until they are validated. Finally, to return to the traditional demand, to engage with the world of the patient with a new onset of jaundice is to appreciate the shock and surprise at the advent of an illness with a range of prognoses from non–life threatening, though painful, gall stones to the insidious progress of malignancy.

To this point, we have been examining the interactions between patients and physicians and their respective sociolects. There are other useful comparisons within the domain of medicine. The advent of illness can dramatically alter the world of being of the patient. Susan Sontag wrote of sickness as becoming a resident of "the kingdom of the ill."[9] The land of illness has its own particular sociolect that shapes the altered reality of the recently immigrated sufferer. Previously simple words such as *future*, *hope*, *vacation*, and *family* take on new shades of meaning not immediately understood by those who are healthy. Visits to the hospital for chemotherapy or radiation treatments are attended by newly realized fears and the institutional buildings may themselves continue to evoke frissons of foreboding even after successful recoveries. This unusual barrier to understanding may heighten the sense of isolation patients sometimes experience and place added demands on physicians, family members, and others who wish to be supportive and helpful. As in all modes of transcultural comprehension, recognition of the issue, a need for attentive listening with the requisite sensibility, and calibrated responses are paramount in gaining understandings of newly acquired meanings.

The shift in world view in moving from the land of the healthy to the land of the ill brings to mind two other experiential reframings. An interesting subtype is found in the diaries and autopathographies of physicians who have themselves experienced severe illnesses and bring back journalistic reports of their travels and travails. In many instances, the stimulus for writing by such caregivers is the recognition of how their understanding of the experience of illness was altered by their own encounters with medicine, this time as recipients of health care. These reports rarely deal with the technical aspects of treatment, such as the decisions for medications or other interventions. They generally describe the isolation, poor communication, and neglect of the humane aspects of care. Physicians as patients speak of the discomfort of their caregivers in coping with the illnesses of colleagues and their own trepidations in feeling at the mercy of a system prone to errors and confusion. Most poignantly perhaps, such narratives describe a new-found, retrospective realization of the experiences of others and the half-remembered stories of patients for whom they provided care—coupled, understandably, with an implicit promise to reframe their clinical attitudes and behaviors.

Medical students also experience a changing world view during education and clinical training, and the idea of identity formation can be found in books and articles on medical schools. Allusions to this change of perspective were noted in the Just a Medical Student aphorism and are evident to medical educators and those who mentor these budding physicians. Early in training, young medical students express clearly their commitments to the care of patients as persons and engage with them as individuals, often regarding them as surrogates for parents and grandparents. They spend time speaking with and listening to their patients and often become their advocates in the hospital or clinic. Students are very enthusiastic about their initial clinical experiences in the middle phase of medical school and are keen to join the club[10] of their role models and teachers. The stresses of contemporary health care, with its emphasis on turnover and episodic care, and the pressures on nascent physicians to conform to the technologized environments of care, may engender distress and disappointments in these young people. They sense a dissonance and tension between their long-held dreams of doctoring and some of what they witness in quotidian medical care. While they certainly describe very wonderful models of caring physicians and teachers, they also report less happy experiences of detached, even inhumane care. This may lead to a decay of aspirations and a surrender to unattractive prospects. Thus, there is a substantial change of understanding in the journey from first-year medical school to graduation, much of it evident in the altered attitudes reflected in the rapidly evolving sociolects of medical students. Nonetheless, as these trainees progress through residency training and become increasingly secure in their new knowledge and skills and comfortable in their emerging identities, the majority remain true to their core beliefs and attitudes and become wonderful role models for the next generation of caregivers.

Clinical Communication

The sociolect that is the lingua franca within a micro-culture provides a particular familiarity and ease of comprehension among members of that communal group. There are, of course, individual differences in idiosyncratic word usage, personal metaphors and tropes, syntax, and prosody. Such variations are evident in comedic mimicry and theatrical impersonations of well-known societal figures. More important for our purposes are the differences between sociolects and the resultant conclusion that all modes of clinical communication between the various micro-cultures we have discussed are, at the very least, instances of translation between and among linguistic enclaves. However, the fact that language is constitutive of individual worlds that persons inhabit and the idiolects they articulate implies that communication is not simply translation but entails acts of interpretation and hermeneutic insights of understanding.

The difference is described in a vignette offered by a senior medical student who served as a medical interpreter for an English-speaking pediatrician and the mother of the young patient, who was an observant Muslim woman and spoke only Arabic. When the medical student translated the doctor's request and question, "Will the mother bring her son back to clinic in a week's time?" the mother's quick response was, "Insh'allah." The student interpreter then said to the pediatrician, "The mother's answer is 'God willing.'" The puzzled pediatrician said, "That's fine, but is that a yes or a no?" The student immediately understood the conundrum and provided the appropriate translation and requisite interpretation, "The mother said 'God willing' and that means yes."

Thus, even an apparently simple, one-word answer may require interpretation rather than simple translation when the interlocutors use words or concepts that are deeply embedded in a particular cultural sociolect. The importance for clinical communication is that, with the small exception of direct facts such as numbers and dates, the preponderance of linguistic interactions, both verbal and embodied, among persons in the patient–physician arena require painstaking interpretive enactments.

One special feature often cited as an important element of clinical skills is that of empathy. We have addressed this notion briefly in the previous chapter and can now enlarge our understanding of empathy in light of the overview of micro-cultures, language, and worlds of being. The traditional invocation of empathy is to step into the shoes of another as a means of identification. This feat cannot be achieved, on at least two grounds. First, as noted previously, worlds of being are unique to the individual and cannot be directly accessed by another. Second, linguistic interpretation and deciphering of texts are necessary to achieve the clinical engagement required for effective processes of diagnosis and therapy. Even with such insightful acts, texts and persons retain a residuum of mystery and hidden meanings that can never be made fully transparent.

Making Up People

We have described the effect that words have on thoughts and how language shapes the worlds in which we live. There is also the more familiar notion that societal norms and fads influence what comes to be seen as desirable, and even healthy. For example, a century ago, a healthy appearance was associated with a body that we would now describe as overweight (or, Rubenesque) and our current description of a healthy habitus would have been regarded as a consumptive look in Victorian England. A parallel example is the poetically lauded alabaster skin that was once a sign of beauty, while today, those who are tanned year-round are envied for their looks. These phenomena of social labeling were likely associated with appearances that signaled wealth and poverty in their specific chronological contexts. This can be understood as a type of social selective pressure that modulates what is considered in or out, cool or square.

There is also an effect of naming and labeling that is not selective, but rather creative. This was described by the philosopher Ian Hacking as "making up people."[11] He developed the concept that devising a category or classification for a type of person may create the possibility to be a person in a particular way—one that did not exist prior to the creation of the newly minted category. An example of interest to us is a survivor of breast cancer. The term *cancer survivor* entered the medical literature in 1985 with the publication of a thoughtful, reflective piece by a young physician describing the course of his own illness and entitled "The Seasons of Survival."[12] There were, of course, those who achieved long-term remissions and even cure following cancer treatment prior to that year—that is, cancer survivors. However, the assignment of the label as formal status made possible a new way of being a person after successful treatment. In some sense, a new species of the genus, patient, was added to the taxonomy of those who are ill. The novel category was taken up readily, most particularly among women who had experienced good responses to treatment for breast cancer. A Google N-gram search revealed that the phrases "cancer survivor" and "breast cancer survivor" are found only rarely prior to 1985 but show an exponential rise in usage after a sharp inflection point in that year. The National Coalition for Cancer Survivorship was founded soon thereafter with a self-professed mission to replace the descriptor *cancer victim* with *cancer survivor*. It has become a major national advocacy and policy development organization that can mobilize over 100,000 persons to a march or demonstration. Most intriguing from the perspective of language is the current ubiquity of the term *cancer survivor* as a mode of identity and self-definition. What explains this rapid growth of a new archetype and the creation of a new way of being in the world? How were such persons "made up?"

A new class does not arise simply because of the coinage of the label. The context must be ripe and ready. In the middle of the twentieth century, cancer was a stigmatized illness, with the diagnosis kept secret, sometimes from patients themselves. The word was uttered with trepidation and foreboding. The image of cancer was the crab with its connotations of inexorable spread, destruction, and imperialist takeovers. This historical framing is depicted articulately in Susan Sontag's *Illness as Metaphor*, which described the antisocial nature of the disease. This spurred the idea of the patient as a cancer victim, which replaced the earlier generation's victims of polio and other infectious ailments. Adding to the patient's sense of loneliness and impending loss was the sense of imputed guilt and blame for lifestyle choices such as smoking and alcohol abuse. In the instance of breast cancer, as we have noted previously, the burden of responsibility was shifted to patients for lack of diligence in breast self-examinations and timely screenings.

Thus, the possibility of a radically different description of a cancer patient intersected with emergent, grass-roots movements for patient advocacy and autonomy, or, at the least, participation in decision-making, guided by the new access to information afforded by the advent of the World Wide Web. The confluence of the contextual social influences found striking resonance among patients who had indeed become literal survivors as a result of continuing improvements in the outcomes of oncological care. Once influential voices in the cancer research and treatment communities called for a model of cancer as a chronic illness, akin to other continuing though manageable conditions, the community of patients was more than ready for a new construct and framing. A cancer survivor emerged as a new way to be a patient hand in hand with the introduction of the appellation. The subsequent institutionalization of the concept in self-help groups, mass marches, and organized political work demonstrated the recursive nature of making up people. That is, the newly emergent ways of being and the persons thus made up began, through their own behaviors, to reshape the novel identity and, concurrently, attracted many patients to fit themselves to the new evolving models. The survivors, especially among women with breast cancer, learned to replace a previously hidden, lonely, and perhaps shameful identity of corporal disfigurement and a loss of femininity with an ethos of exuberant survivorship with an attendant whiff of triumphalism. And why not? After all, the newfound role of survivorship was grounded in part in actual and perhaps unanticipated longevity. The cumulative energy of the newly recruited survivors engendered important networks of support groups, webs of informal advisors, and a salutary sense of solidarity that replaced the former narrative of loneliness and fear. The team spirit channeled into exercise groups, nutritional support circles, and even into dragon boat racing teams that sprouted throughout the developed world with fanciful and proud titles such as Breast Friends Dragon Racing Team and Paddlers in the Pink. This international phenomenon led to the creation of the International Breast Cancer Paddlers' Commission, which coordinates and supports these groups to benefit the physical health and social well-being of survivors. In addition to happy self-interest, these groups aim to raise awareness of the importance of breast cancer research and have spawned a multitude of pink ribbon campaigns, marches, and major philanthropic efforts and both local and national fundraising initiatives. The national organizations have become active in clinical trial development and the promulgation of screening and treatment guidelines. Direct, hands-on service work has been no less important in the effort to support women and families dealing with the daily challenges of treatment and to educate others on the benefits of lifestyle adaptations and awareness of preventive measures such as exercise and dietary changes.

The persons to whom the new classification is applied, and those who take it upon themselves, namely, those made up by the emergent label, do not simply fill the space so created—their actions and decisions reshape and enlarge the class itself, which may thereby attract further adherents. The recursive remolding of the category by persons who are made up and remake themselves was described by Hacking as a "looping effect,"[13] to underscore the interactions between the classification and the people within the class.

The major interactive effect evident in the media was the enlargement of the class to encompass a wide range of activities and actions, including successful government lobbying to provide additional funds for research, advocacy for patient membership on ethics review boards, directed fundraising, and political action against industries thought to produce toxic carcinogens. The self-selected titles expanded from "survivors" to "thrivers" and "breast cancer warriors." Remarkably, the looping effect unfolded very quickly—over the space of a decade or so—as social movements often do, once a tipping point has been achieved. Estée Lauder makeup counters handed out 1.5 million pink ribbons in the fall of 1992, declared "The Year of the Ribbon" by the *New York Times*. It has become the icon of the breast cancer survivors' movement and is now recognized globally.

This wave of attention and visible success was soon followed by a rather different looping effect that questioned and criticized the label "cancer survivor" and all that it brought in its wake. There were patients who bemoaned the movement as pink kitsch and were not at all comforted by nor comfortable with being known as survivors. The concerns and objections of these women are instructive. Many found fault with what they felt was forced membership in what, to them, became a cult of survivorship. The label had become a stereotype with which they did not identify. In a sense, their desire after completion of treatment regimens was to escape from the land of illness, resettle in their former homes, and leave illness behind. The overweening need was for privacy and a desire to forget. Others were disconcerted by the forced cheerfulness and optimism that was at odds with the side effects of chemotherapy and physical disfigurements of surgery. They wished to express their chagrin, fear, and anger, yet the burgeoning survivor groups were unable to accommodate their dissent. Some women felt they were imposters by being regarded as heroes for having survived—outcomes of a process that did not merit special warrior status. Others rejected the notion of war and battle—some concerned with the irony of eventual loss and some with an imposed requirement to conceal the insults to their bodies and identity. Many women viewed all the kitsch and childlike pink objects as infantilizing to themselves and a mockery of those who had not survived.

These paradoxes and tensions in the community of patients are evident in the work of those who have examined the issues empirically. In a study of the perceptions among healthy undergraduate students, cancer survivors were viewed more positively than cancer patients and the former group was also thought to be of stronger character and more heroic. By contrast, a study of patients in Canada found an overwhelming preference for the label "patient" compared with "survivor" among persons with breast or prostate cancer.[14]

Judy Segal, in her paper entitled "Ageism and Rhetoric" adds an interesting dimension to the phenomenon of labeling and the offense of "ageism" that sets the elderly apart. This can only be countered, she notes, by "inclusion ... through a shift from a rhetoric of classification (that is, how we 'make up people') to a rhetoric of identification."[15]

Whether the word *survivor* and the state of being it makes possible are experienced by persons as a state of comfort or its opposite, what is manifestly clear is the dramatic effect of language—indeed, of one word and all that it entails. It is a clear illustration of the ability of language to not only shape our metaphysical homes but even to create a new kind of person together with the newly formed world she inhabits.

3

The Nature of Metaphor

The patient was admitted to the diagnostic service of the academic med-
ical center to assess several puzzling symptoms that had become manifest
over the preceding two years. "Let me see what I can learn from examining
the new patient," said the medical student on the diagnostic team. "We
must review the weight loss of 10 pounds," opined the gastroenterologist,
recommending some special blood tests. "Let's have a look at that strange
heart sound," murmured the cardiologist, donning her stethoscope. "Aha,"
declared the hematologist, "I now see what this means," glancing at the
numbers in the chart. At the end of her stay in hospital, Ms. Jones com-
plained, "I am still in the dark!"

—A Clinical Story

These comments by the physicians (and physician-to-be) share several linguistic characteristics. They are: commonly heard in a hospital setting; metaphoric; similar to phrases used in daily, conventional discourse; and based on the concept that learning, investigating, reviewing, examining, understanding, and knowing (or not) all stem from an overarching linguistic framework that UNDERSTANDING IS SEEING. Such metaphors, according to the *Oxford English Dictionary* (OED), "are figures of speech in which a name or descriptive word or phrase is transferred to an object or action different from, but analogous to, that to which it is literally applicable." Thus, the spoken words—*see, learn, examining* (in the sense of observing), *review, have a look, now see,* and *in the dark*—are all actions or states derived from the root word SEEING and serve to explain (or illuminate) the state of UNDERSTANDING. A more succinct description is that "the essence of metaphor is ... experiencing one kind of thing or experience in terms of another."[1] Stated differently, the abstract concept of UNDERSTANDING can be construed in terms of the action SEEING. The metaphoric work is accomplished when certain features of visual experience are used to explicate the state of comprehension or knowing. Many familiar linguistic expressions in daily use support this connection between understanding and seeing: an illuminating lecture, the light went on, seeing is believing, eye-witness testimony, an obscure explanation, clear as mud, the theory shed light on the data, your diagnosis is insightful, the pathologist clarified the situation, and my perspective reveals a different picture. These expressions are in such frequent use that they may be mistaken as literal discourse, even though they are examples of figurative language. For example, the word *stethoscope* has its etymological origin in the Greek words for "chest" and "seeing," although the actual intent is to listen. Indeed, the original Laennec stethoscope was a solid wooden dowel, hardly suited to vision.

A Brief History of Metaphors

The word *metaphor* derives from two Greek words meaning "to carry beyond" or "to transfer." Aristotle stressed the cognitive function of metaphors in that one could learn something new by deciphering the attributes transferred from source to target. Metaphors were subsequently understood primarily as linguistic ornamentation to embellish style, persuade listeners, and entertain readers and were not regarded by linguists as parts of ordinary language but of the discourse of theater and poetry, of Shakespeare and the Romantic poets. The trope was considered a device of language that offered a translation from the literal to the figurative. By contrast, Fowler, in his 1908 edition of the *King's English*, noted that "almost all words can be shown to be metaphorical when they do not bear a physical meaning"[2] and that metaphors serve to "express mental perceptions, abstract ideas, and complex relations."[3] Nevertheless, his opinion seemed to be the exception, and interest in metaphors waned in the early and mid-twentieth century. The 1970s witnessed a strong revival of interest in the character and role of metaphors, leading to more recent theoretical and empirical research by cognitive linguists on this important aspect of discourse.

Cognitive Metaphors

Cognitive linguists propose that language is the product of large conceptual networks that are represented in neural circuits in the brain whose non-conscious activities make possible thought, comprehension, and expression. Words are not simple labels strung together in sentences but operate in context and setting by tapping into these hyperlinked networks that draw on memory, prior experiences, databanks of acquired information, and learned cultural tropes to evoke accreted meanings that permit deep understanding of a text or conversation. These neural networks, mirrored structurally (and metaphorically) in the contemporary Internet and its search engines, include learned models, frameworks, and elaborations of semantics together with allusions, creative connections, and overlays of personal and cultural history. Words do not evoke simple linear referents in a one-to-one correspondence. Rather, they stimulate large webs of associations via complex networks whose operations result in meaning and understanding.

Metaphors are conceptual, not simple linguistic entities. They are a particular form of association between concepts that enables us to experience and understand one kind of thing in terms of another. While literal thought might expedite an association of reading and book, that is, *within* conceptual domains, figurative thinking represents association *across* conceptual domains, for example, reading and face. Metaphors allow us to adopt some of the attributes of VISION to grasp the notion of UNDERSTANDING. In turn, these conceptual or cognitive metaphors give rise to metaphoric or linguistic expressions, pictures, and even nonverbal actions that reflect the deeper structures from which they spring. Moreover, by hyperlinking seemingly unrelated domains, conceptual metaphors underwrite novel associations between ideas that constitute discovery and creativity. Such deep metaphoric structures shape our reality. They permit us to use grounded and embodied concepts to grasp abstract notions and also elicit extensions and new aspects of existing ideas. Figurative language creates and constitutes the worlds in which we live.

Mapping Metaphors

In the cognitive metaphor the "source" for the properties that are attributed is SEEING and the "target" for these attributions is UNDERSTANDING. By convention, the target and source domains, in this instance, UNDERSTANDING IS SEEING, are noted in small capital letters, to distinguish the basic or root conceptual metaphor from the metaphoric expressions that flow from it, presented in ordinary lower-case letters. An overarching metaphor that provides the grounding for the many actual expressions that are derived from that basic metaphor is referred to as a generic cognitive metaphor. In many instances, source domains are concrete, physical, or readily apparent entities and target domains are abstract, hard-to-grasp ideas. The source domain provides specific descriptors or attributes that help us understand "fuzzy" concepts. Metaphors provide structure for abstractions, ideas, and concepts.

Mapping a metaphor involves an analysis of the relationships between the domains and a tracing of the trajectories of the attributes that flow from the source to the target. Tracking the connections also reveals deeper cognitive links that underpin the basic metaphor and others that derive from it. Thus, the generic cognitive metaphor may give rise to more specific associated metaphors in a hierarchy that shares conceptual features. Finally, in addition to the cardinal aspects of the source transferred to the target, the source domain of the conceptual metaphor may furnish additional attributes that expand range of the original target. These are known as metaphoric entailments or consequences that flow from the underlying cognitive links.

It may be useful to develop these terms and webs of metaphors by using the specific example noted earlier to examine the source and target domains of the conceptual metaphors that share mappings and/or entailments with the basic metaphor UNDERSTANDING IS SEEING (I now *see* what this *means*). The connection between the target and source can be discerned by recalling the common experience that we cannot see things in the dark. Daylight permits examination of our surroundings and affords access to concrete information about the world. This literal state of our being in the world is then reflected in the related metaphors IGNORANCE IS DARKNESS (I'm in the *dark*, the symptom is *obscure*) and its opposite, KNOWLEDGE IS LIGHT (a *bright* idea, I *see* the reason for the pain). An additional basic metaphor relevant to this array is a VISUAL FIELD IS A CONTAINER (I saw her in the *corner of my eye*, the ship came *into view*), a member of a large set for which CONTAINER serves as the source domain. This provides AWARENESS IS VISION (*wake up* and *see the light*) and TO KNOW IS TO SEE (I *know* what I *see*). Perhaps a less common variant is TRUTH IS LIGHT (I *believe* what I *see*; the truth will *come to light*; I do not *see* the need for this vaccine).

By considering VISUAL FIELD IS A CONTAINER in juxtaposition to MIND IS A CONTAINER (this is what I *have in mind*; a *lost* thought; he *lost* his mind), we note a parallel between visual space and mental space, both construed as containers, arriving at IDEAS ARE OBJECTS. Thus, images or percepts are objects in the visual field and the mind is where ideas reside (the plans are in my *head*). The source domain, VISION, of the basic cognitive metaphor UNDERSTANDING IS SEEING is a word with rich allusions and connotations that can themselves serve as sources for new metaphors derived from or entailed by the original construct. Metaphorical entailments result from additional attributions derived from the source domain carried over to aspects of the target domain. Such entailments enrich the array of linguistic metaphors generated from the basic cognitive metaphor. If LIGHTS help us see objects, then INSIGHTS help us decipher ideas (your idea *shines a spotlight* on the problem; the data are a *flash of lightning*; the biopsy was *enlightening*). SHOWING as the sharing of images is a source for sharing of ideas, hence, for COMMUNICATING and teaching (I *showed* the student how to solve the equation). In a similar vein, EXPLICATING IS DRAWING A PICTURE (the circuit *diagram* was *self-explanatory*; the cartoon of the immune system is an *eye-opener*) and a scientific MODEL depicts NOTIONS of causality (the *orrery* helped me *understand* eclipses; the heart is a *pump*). By contrast, yet derived from the same basic construct, is IMPEDIMENTS TO SEEING ARE BARRIERS TO KNOWING (he pulled the wool *over my eyes*; the *fog* of theory). Entailments are of added interest, as the elaboration of networks sprouting from the basic metaphor is a source of originality and creativity. Indeed, CREATIVITY IS SEEING IN A NEW LIGHT (the theory offered a *novel prospect*) and the MIND IS A CONTAINER metaphor give rise to REMEMBERING IS RETRIEVAL (my memory *banks are empty*, false-*memory* syndrome), and in the OED definition of memory we find "the cultural current that looks to loot the baby-boomer memory banks for recyclable cinematic ideas."

The notion that conceptual metaphors are deep cognitive structures (perhaps resident in physical neural networks) stems in part from the prevalence and diversity of common metaphoric expressions. It also gains support from the connections evident in etymology and usage. Etymological unpacking demonstrates that words are themselves the products of old metaphoric connections. This can be illustrated by tracing the linguistic expressions grounded in the UNDERSTANDING IS SEEING cognitive metaphor. The etymological source of *idea* is the Greek word *idein*, "to see," which is related to the Latin *specere*, also "to see or behold." The Latin root is the source of *speculate*, "to observe or view mentally, contemplate, and theorize upon." The word *comprehension* has multiple definitions in the OED: "inclusion," "the faculty of grasping with the mind, power of receiving and containing ideas, mental grasp," and "understanding." These illustrate the reification of ideas contained in the mind and the resultant grasp that constitutes understanding. This concatenation through which ideas are understood as objects is reminiscent of the figurative trope "in the mind's eye." Reflected, one might say, in one of the many OED definitions of the verb *see*: "to perceive (an object, person, scene, etc.) in the mind's eye."

How Do Metaphors Arise?

The metaphoric expressions we have been discussing are readily recognizable and so diverse that we may be tempted to assume that any concrete source can serve any abstract target. Yet, that is clearly not the case. For example, "a sharp mind" seems to fit, it is congruent with our sense of the world, while "an upholstered mind" seems to us askew. So how and where do metaphors arise and what does it mean for a metaphor to fit, to seem right?

Metaphors are rooted in three types of human experience: perceptual, biological, and cultural. Visual metaphors are common and stem from the notion that we experience the world through our senses, of which vision is considered to be the most important mode of acquiring information about our surroundings. Perceptions come in through our eyes, resulting in the container cognitive metaphors of the visual field and the mind (brain), with an intake conduit via the retina. Another group of experiential metaphors termed *orientational* refer to the common concepts of spatial arrangements. The biological fact that humans are upright animals, together with common experiences in the world, results in the primary metaphors of MORE IS UP and LESS IS DOWN. Presumably, watching a lake fill with water during a rainstorm conjures up an association between more material and an upward sweep in the visual field. This primary metaphor derives directly from human experience. What connects MORE and UP is not a perceived linguistic similarity or synonymy between the two words, but rather an experiential correlation between the two. That is, more water in the lake leads to a horizon shifting upward. High blood pressure is signaled by a rising column of mercury in a traditional sphygmomanometer. If we sense a whiff of synonymy between MORE and UP, it is due to the embeddedness of the metaphor and its influence on our thoughts, rather than a pre-existing similarity. The distinction demonstrates that metaphors are not grounded in literal linguistic similarities but in cognitive correlations and connections derived from experience and subsequently generalized to further linkages. We refer to the growth of money, the decline of the stock market, and upwardly mobile neighbors—all grounded in the orientational metaphor. Less directly, HAPPINESS IS UP (she's on *cloud nine*) and SADNESS IS DOWN (he's in the *dumps*) rely on the primary orientational metaphors and a biological response in which the emotion of happiness leads to a feeling of lightness, a sense of buoyancy, and an upright gait. By contrast, depression correlates with a desire to sleep, a choice of darkness, and a slack physical posture. Metaphors rooted in biology often reflect bodily states and sensations and indicate that many common metaphors result from human experiences gained through our senses and interactions with the lived environment.

Metaphors, like all language, are rooted in culture and reflect social frames and tropes. The classical humoral model of medicine viewed illness as the result of imbalances among the four humors: phlegm, black bile, yellow bile, and blood. While these traditional notions are no longer used in Western medicine to explain the pathogenesis of disease, words and metaphors based on them remain. The sanguine personality, a bilious disposition, and a melancholic mood are direct metaphoric descendants of the humoral theory and also evident in many linguistic expressions (the patient is *out of sorts*, he's *off his rocker*, a *temperamental* child, an *unbalanced* mind). The idea of balance, or homeostasis, remains a predominant frame in traditional Chinese medicine and was a mainstay of physiology in Euro-American science in the mid-twentieth century. Homeostasis as a trope, however, has been largely supplanted in Western medicine by the BODY IS A MACHINE and the MIND IS A COMPUTER cognitive metaphors. The former provides the expressions he suffered a total *breakdown*, she is *out of gas*, I *blew a gasket*, he is a *sparkplug,* and the latter is reflected in he needs to be *reprogrammed*, a need to *reboot,* and his *software* is buggy. Prevalent metaphors depend on contemporary cultural ideas and are rooted in theories of explanation dominant at a given time and place. In addition to the source domain of COMPUTER to understand the MIND, highlighting calculating power and logic, older sources have included a TELEPHONE EXCHANGE, alluding to communication, crossed wires, and connectivity; a HYDRAULIC PUMP, drawing attention to the flow of ideas and an overflowing dam; and a DARK WEB, emphasizing mystery, unpredictability, and a barrier to self-knowledge. Metaphors and language are archival remnants of the historical flow of concepts and once-prevalent ideas about the world shared by societies. This accumulation of evolving tropes and their associated connotations led Alice Deignan to refer to metaphoric expressions as "a cultural reliquary."[4] In turn, each particular culture and the meanings it creates is shaped by the language and metaphors it inherits. These webs of significance embedded in language inflect and shape the thoughts of its speakers, as contemplated by Whorf and Sapir.

The transfer of attributes from source to target is selective, as are the aspects of the target that are highlighted. The source COMPUTER points to the ability of the MIND to conduct logical processes but ignores or hides the capacity to forget that is the focus of the MIND IS CONTAINER metaphor. This highlighting–hiding selectivity of attention accounts for the rhetorical power of metaphors—the speaker can direct the listener toward certain features while submerging others. This capacity also explains why highly abstract and complex targets are often linked to a variety of sources, each pointing to a different feature (much like the parable of the blind men and the elephant). Conversely, sources have a variety of qualities and properties—some are used to characterize the target while others are not salient. The CONTAINER as source for the targets VISION and MIND highlights space and capacity (visual field and memory register) but neither the shape of the container nor the material from which it is made are deemed relevant. Thus, the accord between the two domains is partial, rather than complete. And, the same source domain, for example, CONTAINER can be associated with many different targets. It is therefore more useful to describe TARGET *as* SOURCE rather than TARGET *is* SOURCE, the latter implying complete congruence. These properties make possible the rich web of connectivity across and among many conceptual domains. They point to the polysemous nature of metaphor and its powerful allusiveness and, at times, elusiveness in highlighting certain aspects of the target while diverting attention from others.

How does a metaphor fit and how does it make sense? A partial answer comes from an intuition that the selected attributions from SOURCE to TARGET are in accord with our experience, expectations, and shared cultural knowledge and values. When a scientist says that a given theory is worthy of pursuit or a model of a gene is beautiful, what is being expressed is not a logical conclusion of proof but rather a coherence with expectations and an intuitive sense of rightness. The theory proposed may be a radical disruption of a prior picture or model and its attractiveness may arise from the dramatic novelty and a gut feeling of validity. In other settings, fitness of a metaphor is dependent on culture and context. Certain models of the good life value harmony while others opt for victory. For example, the predominant tradition in business negotiation has been for each party to seek victory in a winner-takes-all outcome—an instance of the NEGOTIATION IS WAR metaphor. This is so engrained in our culture that when individuals working to negotiate peaceful coexistence proposed a process they called *Getting to Yes* as a win-win model, it was hailed as a novelty. A new metaphor that NEGOTIATION IS A DANCE is likely strange to us yet may express a normative value in a different cultural setting.

A study of the seasonal variation in the prevalence of linguistic expressions of the source domain HEALTH in editorials in the *Economist* illustrates the influence of context. An enumeration of expressions such as "*sickly* firms . . . a *chronic* deficit . . . a financial *injection*"[5] by months of the year revealed an almost two-fold greater appearance of such metaphors in the winter months (in England) compared with the summer season. Winter is a time of respiratory illnesses and feelings of malaise, increasing the salience of such embodied linguistic expressions. The editorialists themselves may not have been aware of this seasonal fluctuation in utilization, underscoring that linguistic games often take place in the mental backgrounds of our unconscious selves. The influence of context illustrates the embeddedness of cognitive metaphors in changing conditions of experience, whether seasonal, cultural, or physical, as well as the inseparability of body and mind.

Metaphors are a common occurrence in discourse and writing. This is, of course, in contrast to an older perception that figurative language is found primarily in poetry and literary texts. Studies reveal that metaphoric words and expressions are used quite liberally in daily speech and writing. Pollio and colleagues[6] surveyed the speech of politicians in public and of therapists speaking with patients and found an average of five figures of speech per one hundred spoken words. They estimated that the reader of fiction will encounter three figures per page of text, school textbooks

present a 1 percent rate of occurrence of figures of speech, and an eleventh-grade student will read an average of five figures per page. A detailed and careful study examined a large body of words from actual English discourse, both written and spoken.
A metaphor was identified in 13.6 percent of the words in the sample—once every
7.5 words—a surprisingly high number! The frequency varied from 18.5 percent in
academic writings to 7.7 percent in conversation. Expression in spoken and written
language evidently requires metaphors. The dependence of communication on metaphor is found, perhaps paradoxically, at the beginning of Susan Sontag's influential
book, *Illness as Metaphor*. Sontag articulated a passionate demand for clear, literal
language to describe the impact of illness—yet, the first sentence of the text is highly
figured and invokes a novel metaphor on the state of patienthood. "Illness is the night-
side of life," Sontag tells us, "a more onerous citizenship. Everyone who is born holds
dual citizenship, in the kingdom of the well and in the kingdom of the sick. Although
we all prefer to use only the good passport, sooner or later each of us is obliged, at
least for a spell, to identify ourselves as citizens of that other place."[7] The apparent
discrepancy between the prevailing sense that metaphors are used infrequently in ordinary discourse and the empirical findings of their ubiquity may be due to the oxymoron of the literal metaphor. Many figures of speech have become so common that
they have become conventional means to describe abstract ideas. The passage of time,
an explosion of energy, an uphill battle, a quest for justice—these figures of speech,
among many others, are so engrained that their use has become accepted as literal
and conventional. They have even been described as dead metaphors, thus hinting at
the subtle influence of metaphors on how we experience the world.

Literal, nonfigurative language is linear, clear, and constrained. To foster clarity
and avert misunderstandings, words are chosen to avoid multiple interpretations, as
in an instruction manual for an appliance or a legal contract. What is sacrificed is the
novelty that stems from open-ended possibilities and the creativity of as-yet unimag-
ined associations. Metaphoric connections involve abstract concepts that are illuminated by characteristics drawn from one or more source domains. In turn, a given
source domain may furnish useful properties for several target domains, otherwise
unassociated with one another. The result is a branching or arborescent web across
multiple conceptual domains, affording many pathways to new associations that constitute creative thinking. The capacity to spur the generation of novel ideas is characteristic of scientific theories and models, often described as fruitful. To cite a famous
example: selective breeding of animals and plants to improve agricultural produc-
tivity is an accepted practice that is also pursued by various hobbyists, such as pigeon
fanciers and orchid growers. This methodology was widespread long before the underlying genetic mechanisms were deciphered and understood and served as a source
concept for the development of eugenics towards the end of the nineteenth century.
The same source domain provided a metaphoric extension that Charles Darwin applied to explain the data he had gathered over many decades demonstrating the evolution of species. Breeding and directed, intentional selection provided the model for
the mechanism of natural selection as the explanatory framework for the evolution of

species and the descent of humankind. The insight was certainly revolutionary and a shift of historical paradigms for the origin of species—yet it stemmed from prior metaphoric models understood in novel ways by prepared eyes! Thus, the ancient techniques of animal husbandry are projected metaphorically onto the data of natural philosophy to generate a dramatic realignment in science and culture.

While metaphoric entailments that contribute to linguistic novelty may seem at first to simply offer a new mode of expression or description, a more careful review indicates that figurative language makes possible and also mirrors and perhaps underlies intellectual discovery. Metaphors are potent linguistic objects that represent abstract ideas and make them tangible by giving them a semblance of concreteness. They thereby become available to manipulation by thinking and reasoning. Mental games, that is, language games, use metaphoric elements that can be realigned, mixed, and shuffled and connected along pathways afforded by the networks and webs of allusions and their cross-domain links. These games result not simply in new words but instantiate novel ideas. Metaphors make possible an understanding of abstractions, and their reassortments constitute reasoning and creativity. Words frame and reframe our perceptions and thoughts to permit us to see what was heretofore unknown. Perhaps paradoxically, the sciences abound in figurative language. For example, theoretical physicists, who pride themselves in precision, seek to understand the cosmos through abstractions made accessible by metaphoric models that speak of strings, waves, particles, and Schrodinger's cats—all thoroughly figurative yet rich in predictions later confirmed by empirical means. The need to deal in abstractions may explain the high prevalence of metaphors in academic discourse, even in the natural sciences.

Framing Reality

The rich webs of ideas crafted by metaphors permit abstract reasoning, creative insights, and perhaps learning and intellectual development. This is the constitutive power of language, not simply its capacity to reveal. Reality as such is not reshaped, but our perceptions, experiences, and our worlds of being are certainly framed and experienced through language. Not surprisingly, words are not neutral. Metaphors shift our gaze and act selectively—they have their own capacity to constrain. If the linguistic expression "the light suddenly went on" helps us deal with ideas as objects, it also entails that we understand ideas all at once. That is quite fine for an idea as image, such as a picture or cartoon, but undermines the concept of the gradual accretion of understanding acquired slowly and painstakingly through interpretive study. The metaphor of enlightenment, coupled with our contemporary fondness for instant communication, is, perhaps paradoxically, antithetical to thoughtful reasoning and analysis. Similarly, the ubiquitous metaphor of the BODY IS MACHINE directs caregivers to consider oil changes and replacements of parts in managing chronic ailments and the MIND IS COMPUTER creates an expectation of rapid solutions and supports the current hyper-speed of quick medical encounters aided by machines in the consulting room.

This property of selectivity, or, highlighting and hiding, characteristic of metaphors led one scholar to coin the term "transformative symbolic structures,"[8] noting that metaphors reshape our picture of reality, referring to them as "co-authors of our reality."[9] Language transforms our sense of what is real—the domain of facts—and shapes our beliefs of what is important—the domain of values.

Language, Discourse, Culture, and Concepts

Metaphors that stem from embodied experiences, such as HAPPY IS UP, are generally universal and transcend particular languages. In other instances, metaphors in one country use source domains familiar to that society that are less salient in other settings. Metaphors in Britain often draw on sailing, gardening, and horse racing, while French discourse reflects an interest in food and cuisine, and Spanish privileges bullfighting. The Italian word for "mouth" appears in metaphors for eating, while in English it more often is associated with speaking. There is then a two-way interaction between metaphors and cultural tropes common in a given society or its subgroups. Novel metaphors spread through daily discourse and may become part of idiomatic expressions in common use. These are then learned by newcomers to the language, whether through immigration or birth, and become part of the evolving cultural heritage. Tropes that remain embedded over long spans of time may become conventionalized while retaining their power to direct attention and shape reality. Such metaphors are linguistically powerful as they influence our thinking and perceptions in a manner that is below our immediate awareness. A current example is the power of an old notion that bacteria are harmful invaders, which makes it difficult to accept the concept of the microbiome and the necessity of bacteria for human function and integrity. Linguistic tropes are utilized in daily dialogue and are evoked routinely to communicate content. At the same time, the particular choices made by the speaker are accompanied by accreted attitudes, values, and emotions.

Language, Thought, and Being

Language shapes our thinking, inflects our reality, and defines our values and attitudes—in a word, language makes us who we are. The work of Carol Cohn, a feminist scholar who carried out a yearlong ethnographic study of the habits and discourse of defense planners in the United States, illustrates the concepts developed in this chapter.

The planners, whether from the academy or government, were persons of good will who saw themselves working within a rational framework. At the same time, their subject of interest was nuclear warfare, weaponry, and deterrence, whose destructive power entails the loss of millions of lives within a few minutes or hours. How then did such persons cope rationally with the potential for total destruction? Cohn observed a shift from direct descriptive language to one of abstractions, euphemisms, metaphors, and acronyms. Language became a means of obscuring the truth and providing distance from reality. Common terms were "clean bombs" (rather than nuclear weapons) that are "delivered" (rather than dropped), by "damage limitation vehicles" (rather than missiles), in "counter-value attacks" (rather than bombing cities), causing "collateral damage" (rather than human casualties). "Surgically clean strikes,"[10] a metaphor whose source domain is SURGERY, promotes an image of an aseptic bombing attack, ostensibly good for your health. These sanitizing abstractions of "words so bland that they never forced the speaker or enabled the listener to touch the realities of nuclear holocaust that lay behind the words"[11] created "an astounding chasm between image and reality" that enabled the requisite detachment and diminished affect. Otherwise, "to be accountable to reality is to be unable to do this work."

In addition to whitewashing reality, figurative language provided (black) humor and redirected attention. The focal point of discussions became the weapons themselves, whose power was admired and celebrated. As Cohn described, "there simply is no way to talk about human death or human societies when you are using a language designed to talk about weapons." Persons are no longer part of the discourse and disappear when the special language renders them irrelevant. The talk of the strategic experts had further benefits—the arcane, insiders' language created a bond among the experts, a "nuclear priesthood,"[12] that excluded others not fluent in the argot. The insiders enjoyed "the thrill of being able to manipulate an arcane language, the power of entering the secret kingdom, being someone in the know."[13]

Cohn found that to engage the defense intellectuals in any discussions of the impact and implications of their work necessitated that she learn to speak the language. Otherwise, she was regarded as an outsider. "What I found was that no matter how well-informed or complex my questions were, if I spoke English rather than expert jargon, the men responded to me as though I were ignorant, simpleminded, or both."[14] Once she learned and adopted the discourse and its tropes, she no longer found them strange, and "speaking the language, I could no longer hear it. . . . I had not only learned to speak a language; I had started to think in it. Its questions became my questions, its concepts shaped my responses to new ideas. Its definitions of the parameters of reality became mine."[15] Cohn suddenly realized that learning and using the new language entailed a new mindset and perceptual framework, inviting "the transformation, the militarization, of our own thinking."[16] As she noted, "I found that my own thinking was changing,"[17] and "the language shapes your categories of thought."[18]

What explains the allure of a new language with its rather potent effects? In the case of the nuclear strategic thinkers, there are the previously mentioned benefits of distance from otherwise difficult concepts of death and destruction and of membership in an inner circle. Cohn observed that the latter provides two added attractions: a sense of power that follows knowing what only few others share and the attendant feeling of control. As she points out: "Few know, and those who do are powerful. You can rub elbows with them, perhaps even be one yourself.... A more subtle ... element of learning the language is that when you speak it, you feel in control.... You can get so good at manipulating the words that it almost feels as though the whole thing is under control."[19]

However, the new adept may soon realize that the price of admission is significant. There is the risk of entrapment in the new discourse. "I began to find it difficult to get out" and "You become subject to the tyranny of concepts" were two of many such observations. More significant is the loss of previous understandings: "My grasp on what I knew as reality seemed to slip,"[20] and the new language provided different "parameters of reality [that] became mine," so that "the content of what you can talk about is monumentally different." The altered mindset was experienced by the ethnographer without prior intent or desire and seemed to parallel the linguistic change itself.

The process that attends the acquisition of the novel discourse and metaphors is not a conscious choice of detachment or dampened sensibilities. Rather, it necessarily follows the enculturation into the language and its framing of the world. This change of identity is a "transformative, rather than an additive, process."[21] It may proceed gradually but there seems to be an inflection point en route when one views the world through different lenses.

Language in the Clinical Setting

This striking example of the interface among language, context, and mindset is mirrored in a similarly intense, closed, and jargon-laden setting, the clinical environment. Acronyms, metaphors, and a cryptic language characterize the discursive environment of doctors and patients and shape the emotional tone of the clinical relationship. A medical student first encountering the tropes of hospital parlance may learn to describe a patient as "the gall bladder admitted this morning who claims to have three days of abdominal pain" without realizing that the first part of that phrase is a metonymy (or synecdoche) in which the name of the suspect organ substitutes for the patient. (Metonymy is a figure of speech that is a comparison within a single domain, rather than across domains characteristic of a metaphor). The use by the student of the engrained and perhaps conventionalized trope may be quite innocent yet results in a depersonalization of the patient whose presence is deemed irrelevant by the attention directed to the inflamed gall bladder. The second segment using the word "claims" casts a shadow of doubt on the patient's description by avoiding the direct language that the patient had three days of abdominal pain. After all, how do we know the patient's report is accurate? Thus, the medical phrase is hedged with the language of a claim to land or an insurance claim—both are tentative until confirmed. Once again, the student is unintentionally discounting the words and authority of the patient as speaker by absorbing the tropes of the medical guild.

Students are socialized, gradually assume their identities, and join the club of care-givers by learning the discourse and cultural mores of the profession. Even as this is appropriate and necessary, when the language witnessed by the young students is laden with pejorative metaphors whose impact may not be immediately apparent to the learners, and perhaps not even to the clinical mentors who serve as role models, then the hidden tropes are not salutary but insidious. They may intoxicate the clinical environment. Educators Cameron and Low observed that participants in a conversation may use metaphors to broach an uncomfortable subject, such as commenting negatively about a third party.[22] The use of figurative, indirect language permits the interlocutors to make common cause with each other while distancing themselves from a difficult situation. This has the unfortunate effect of unidimensionally trivial-izing their opponents, leading to disengagement from direct patient contact. Joining the club of clinicians, the medical student assumes a measured remove from the dis-comfort of caring for (and about) a complex patient and thus disengages from the duties and obligations to the person who is ill. Little wonder that medical students describe a dissonance and tension between their aspirations as nascent physicians and the detachment they discern in the behaviors and language of their role mod-els. They feel the undertow of these submerged metaphors, unaware that their angst stems from the discourse they are learning, even as it provides entry to the club they yearn to join.

To be sure, one goal of education is personal transformation, and becoming a health care professional is to undergo metamorphosis. What is particularly inter-esting is that one major pathway of change is the acquisition of new metaphors and other figurative tropes—indeed, a novel language. An important corollary to the con-cept of transformation via linguistic enculturation is that responsibility for the con-sequences, be they good or ill, should not be ascribed to individuals alone. Figurative language emanates from a deep and broad cultural and historical context. It is the outcome of extended periods of cultural evolution and selection with novelty intro-duced by linguistic interbreeding and technological demands. The resultant language inflects perception and shapes choices. It shifts our attention and infuses our values and attitudes. While it is indeed the case that individual persons make judgments and choices, the actual outcomes are contingent on many contextual factors, not least among them being the languages we acquire and that resonate within us.

II

THE MILITARY METAPHORS
OF MEDICINE

4
The Militarized Arena of Medicine

Barack Obama ... when he learned that McCain had been diagnosed with cancer, commented: "Cancer doesn't know what it's up against."
—The Guardian Obituary

The brain-cancer diagnosis in July 2017 freed his tongue, and tested his mettle, in all the ways he relished.
—The Economist Obituary

Legendary senator John McCain has died after a nearly year-long bout with glioblastoma, a form of brain cancer.
—Rolling Stone Obituary

The suggestion that the predominant metaphor in the discourse of medicine is that of war and the military is generally met with puzzlement and skepticism. This trope is common in both formal and casual speech and writings of health care professionals, patients, and journalists, and yet most are unaware of its ubiquity. In actuality, such figures of speech are only too common in the daily language of medicine in hospitals and clinics and in the public arena. Franklin Roosevelt launched the March of Dimes campaign against poliomyelitis; Richard Nixon announced a war on cancer; Lyndon Johnson extended the idea to public health with a war on poverty; Bill Clinton's administration fought a war on drugs; and Barack Obama and Joe Biden reignited the continuing war on cancer with a "moonshot plan" to conquer the disease. American presidents defined important social policy agendas in terms of battles to be fought and foes to be vanquished. We speak heroically of eradicating infectious diseases caused by our enemies—bacteria and viruses—and other agents of disease. Oncologists fight fire with fire as tumors are locally invasive, aggressive, silent, and widespread or under control—metaphoric descriptors consonant with an imperialist, militarized view of malignancy. The requisite therapeutic array is a repository of weaponry that can extirpate, poison, and burn tumors in guerilla warfare that entails collateral damage to bystander healthy cells. Operating rooms are theaters, and emergency rooms, known in England as casualty units, are sites of triage. We are told to eat well to strengthen the body's defenses, in preparation for the battle against infections, to avert heart attacks and sidestep immune cells that turn against our bodies. Of course, to win, we must follow doctors' orders and never give up the good fight.

In the clinical setting, the discourse is similarly replete with images of war with its outcomes of victory or loss. Infections overwhelm and are treated with shotgun therapy, tumors infiltrate and are treated aggressively, defenses are breached and need to be shored up, and diagnostic assessments are launched with a battery of laboratory tests and imaging procedures. This mindset is reflected in the titles of health care personnel. Young physicians in hospital training are house officers and the nation's top public health doctor is the Surgeon General with the rank of Vice-Admiral in the United States Public Health Service Commissioned Corps.

The general public is also urged to join the fight against disease. In 1936, the General Federation of Women's Clubs proposed a legion of volunteers "to wage war on cancer,"[1] known as The Women's Field Army.[2] Its recruits wore khaki uniforms, with insignia of military rank and implemented a highly successful campaign to raise money and educate the public-at-large. This followed soon after the profession's declarations of war. In a lead editorial in 1934, entitled "The War Against Cancer," the *British Medical Journal* discussed the "world-wide campaign against cancer" noting that "cancer, *if taken in time*, is frequently amenable to treatment[3]" (italics in original text), with a laudatory review of a volume with the title *La Lutte Internationale Contre le Cancer*. The rhetoric, in both professional and public arenas, gained in energy and force. The Women's Field Army "war cry"[4] demanded "trench warfare with a vengeance against a ruthless killer," while scholarly publications called for "a carefully planned military campaign" that necessitated an "increase [in] the caliber of our weapons."[5] Politicians joined the fray as then Senator Olympia Snowe demanded that we "wage war against a brutal and merciless enemy: breast cancer."[6]

The war metaphor was commonplace on websites of major organizations dedicated to health care. Sloan-Kettering displayed its research program as "Finding New Ways to Conquer Cancer"; the American Cancer Society asked us to see how we're attacking cancer from every angle and its traditional radio ads invited the public to fight cancer with a check-up and a check; the American Stroke Association informed us that stroke is beatable; and the Alzheimer's Association exhorted us to become volunteers by announcing that "together, we are stronger! Explore the many ways to join the fight against Alzheimer's disease." Another index of the use of combative language is evident in the titles of popular books for patients with cancer and their families. Cookbooks sport titles such as *The Cancer Fighting Kitchen,* and *Recipes to Fight Disease,* and traditional self-help books are promoted with such titles as *90 Days to Live: Beating Cancer When Modern Medicine Offers No Hope,* and *Cancer Secrets: An Integrative Oncologist Reveals How You Can Defeat Cancer Using the Best of Modern Medicine and Alternative Therapies.* The official history of the American Cancer Society is entitled *Crusade.*

If the war metaphor is ubiquitous, why then the puzzlement when this observation is offered? This powerful trope is so deeply engrained in our rhetoric and culture that it has become accepted as simple descriptive language. We have lost sight of the influence and impact of this metaphor on our thoughts and behaviors. The militaristic origins of the words and ideas we often use to understand, explain, and make sense of disease and illness deeply shape communication among the participants in medicine and health.

To understand why such tropes have influence and to decipher their effects, both good and ill, we ask: Who is fighting whom, and why? Who are the winners and losers? What does conquest entail, and who is the victim? Who are the heroes, and who is responsible for defeats?

Doctor versus Disease

The military or war metaphor in medicine uses the source domains of wars, battles, and military, pugilistic, and antagonistic encounters more generally, to characterize the broad target domain of medicine. This extensive domain encompasses our conceptions of the etiology and pathogenesis of illness and disease, and the acts of assessment, diagnosis, therapy, and management—in short, all aspects of the care of patients. The military frame extends to biomedical research, medical philanthropy, patients' identities and images of themselves, and to the families that provide care and support. The metaphor influences the interactions between individual physicians and their patients as well as the organization of preventive care and public health. It inflects how physicians understand and act out their mandated roles and how the public views and understands disease, illness, and health care. This is not surprising given our understanding that medicine is culturally embedded and culture, in turn, is enacted in language.

Since the war metaphor points to a battle, it requires a protagonist and an enemy. The most common variety is a construct in which the physician is the combatant and disease is the arch-enemy to be vanquished. This model is evident in the therapeutic armamentarium of the physician with its silver bullets, cobalt bombs, and blockbuster biologicals among the great variety of weapons provided by the pharmaceutical industry, and the discoveries by biomedical scientists whose mission is to conquer disease. The enemy may be the disease, the bacteria and viruses as causal agents or the cells that comprise a malignant tumor. The scientist who discovers the bacteria and viruses that are the enemies is a hunter, depicted as a hero in the *Microbe Hunters*,[7] a popular science book of the 1930s. The individual physician searching for the cause of illness of a specific patient is often depicted in the popular media as a Sherlock Holmesian figure who uses diagnostic clues to find the culprit. Though the consulting detective is not per se a military persona, he is mirrored in the search-and-destroy missions of clinical specialists in infectious diseases. Similarly, public health epidemiologists react to outbreaks of serious diseases as members of emergency response teams from the Centers for Disease Control and Prevention (CDC), which works 24/7 "to protect America from health, safety and security threats, both foreign and in the U.S.… CDC fights disease and supports communities and citizens to do the same to protect America from health and safety threats, both foreign and domestic."[8]

The physician in charge is the commander responsible for overall strategy. He—more often than she, for this model tends to be male-dominant—directs the intelligence and spy corps who search to identify the agents responsible. Such experts may include radiologists and imaging specialists, clinical pathologists and microbiologists, and, increasingly, computer scientists who bring to bear the capabilities of artificial intelligence. The surgeon- or physician-general is also the tactical commander of the war to conquer the disease, a fighter whose allies are the quartermaster in charge of the blood bank, the anesthesiologist providing sedation, and the radiation oncologist marshaling the radiotherapy machines.

This metaphoric construction is accompanied by significant entailments. In this bilateral militarized relationship between the doctor and the disease, what then is the role assigned to the person who is suffering? Prefigured by the sources of the word *patient* from the Latin root for "suffering" and attendant meanings of tolerance and passivity, the ill person is the battleground on which the war is fought. This figure of the doctor as protagonist, together with a traditional paternalistic mode of medical practice, does not provide space for consultations with the patient as an ally in the fight and renders that person as a passive, perhaps anesthetized, field of war. This perhaps unintended, yet significant, transformation of the patient into an inanimate and unengaged landscape of battle is at odds with contemporary ideas of patients as decision makers and autonomous agents who make health care choices on the advice of physicians. It undermines a collaborative alliance between doctors and their patients and renders patients mute. It may also explain the oft-heard complaint that surgeons do not talk with their patients. After all, a general may inspect the configuration of the field of battle on the evening before attack—he is, however, not likely to ask for its opinions!

The physician's attention is directed to the disease, whether as a puzzle to be solved by astute diagnostics or an enemy to be defeated by potent therapeutics. The medical gaze is deflected from the purported object of health care, the ailing patient who has come seeking help, to the disease that becomes the hill to be conquered. The disease is reconfigured from an abnormal process of pathophysiology to an independent entity. The disease is reified and what was abstract becomes a concretized object that can be sought, found, attacked, and destroyed. This transformation may indeed help capture and focus the energy of the physician. However, the shift renders the patient as a vessel bearing a reified disease or a mode of transport bringing the disease to the physician's attention. Thus, the object of care becomes, for example, a pneumonia, rather than a person afflicted by a bacterial infection of the lungs. In the former instance, all pneumococcal pneumonias are pretty much alike, while in the latter formulation, each person exhibits a somewhat idiosyncratic process of illness. Indeed, the former is a disease, separate from specifics, while the latter is an illness whose manifestations and import depend on context of person, place, and time. Lastly, pneumonia as the disease is treated somewhat generically with an antibiotic, while the patient with an infection of the lungs requires customized treatments with fluids, support, oxygen, and informative explanations, directive consent, and personal attention. There is little doubt that antibiotics are appropriate and necessary in both framings—yet, only the image that illness is a composite reality experienced by a specific person with an underlying physiological and/or psychological process leads necessarily to individualized, person-specific modalities of care. Furthermore, this mindset enables interactions and interventions that are attended by due regard and respect for the dignity of the person who is ill.

Whether the patient has become a battlefield or the vessel bearing disease, the person has become incidental to the object of interest to the physician. In a strange way, the term *incidentaloma*, currently used colloquially to describe an unanticipated finding in an imaging procedure unrelated to the original diagnostic search, can now be applied to the patient, who is a passive bystander or a carrier for the lesion of actual interest to the physician.

In this variant of the war metaphor, in which the physician aims to conquer disease, much like St. George slaying the dragon, who are the winners, the losers, and the victims? In a Western and American cultural frame, evident in movies, television, and other expressions of identity, the archetypal hero is male and often a cowboy or soldier. In the former case, the Wild West is tamed and in the latter, the enemy is defeated. In the medical sphere, when the disease is eliminated by extirpation, whether by surgery, antibiotics, or other interventions, then the physician is both winner and hero. Such a victory may result from the removal of a stone or the setting of a fracture. Even in the setting of mental illness, once thought to be due to psychic invasions by demons or spirits, a psychiatric exorcism is also a form of victory by extirpation. Of course, many illnesses are not susceptible to such metaphoric understandings. One can hardly cut out blood pressure to treat hypertension or remove the immune system to conquer systemic lupus erythematosus. Nonetheless, even in such instances of chronic illness, the modality of control has replaced complete victory to achieve a sort of medical truce! One might expect that the illnesses of aging would be framed in non-aggressive language—nonetheless, we have alluded to campaigns to defeat Alzheimer's disease. In short, whatever the intervention, the physician claims victory and perhaps heroic status when the disease has been removed, eliminated, or forced to a stand-off in a long-lasting truce.

The situation is rather different when things do not go well—and the battle is lost. If the physician is forced to retreat in the face of an overwhelming disease, one might guess that the protagonist-doctor accepts the loss. After all, if you wish to claim credit for winning, should you not accept responsibility for defeat? Yet the language and metaphors used in such settings reveal a rather different picture. A phrase often overheard in oncology settings is that the patient failed drug X and an alternative approach will be used. Or, the general wording, the patient failed chemotherapy, which signals an important shift of therapeutic strategies. These words attribute to the patient the responsibility and blame for the loss. In the first model of war metaphor, the physician-general chooses the strategy and, by implication, claims responsibility for the results. That physician is quite willing to accept kudos for good outcomes and victory. When a loss is imminent, the focus of agency shifts dramatically and the heretofore passive patient learns that he failed a crucial test or trial. When the actual outcomes are those desired by the physician and (usually) the patient, the doctor is the victor and the disease is the victim and loser. When the disease turns out to be a victorious enemy, the patient suddenly becomes the victim and faces a double loss—the agony of defeat and the insult of blame.

A sad reminder of such linguistic turns of phrase is the oft-cited phrase in obituary notices that the person passed away after a valiant or courageous battle with cancer or some other grave disease. Or, a physician or nurse consoling a family might note that a close relative was a tough fighter. Of course, in both instances, the unspoken segue is that the loved one lost the battle. What then should be the status of the non-victorious physician, if not that of loser? To be fair, there are many reasons why interventions and treatments fail to achieve the desired result. The course of illness, the nature of partial or ineffective therapies, and a multitude of contextual factors can contribute to an unfortunate result. The issue at hand is not whether the doctor is free of all responsibility for a less than salutary outcome. What should concern us is the inappropriate attribution of blame and responsibility to the innocent patient. If indeed there are many factors that contribute to a loss, why transform the patient into the blameworthy victim? Parenthetically, we often use the word *victim* to describe a person suddenly afflicted with a serious illness—for example, a victim of polio or AIDS or measles. Thus, if we effectively absolve the physician, surely the patient deserves no less.

Physicians may sometimes signal an intention to retreat from a losing situation with the sad and rather egregious phrase, I am afraid there is nothing more we can do. Yet, there is always something to be offered, even when cures become difficult or impossible. Attention to quality of life, control of symptoms, and alleviation of suffering are no less within the mandate and mission of physicians and medicine than an intent and desire to cure. Many families have remarked that some oncologists are uncomfortable when the goals shift from cure to care and even more so when what is needed is palliative care. Too many cancer doctors stop making visits to their patients who move to late stages of illness and end-of-life care. Perhaps this is a sign of the physicians' own sense of guilt and a lingering responsibility. We may speculate that a shared responsibility between physician and patient crafted at the very initial phases of illness and care would avoid both a heroic physician upon victory and a feeling of loss by either when matters evolve poorly. Perhaps there can be a common understanding by a physician and patient who accept victories and share joy with humility, weather losses with sanguinity, and share commitments for the full course of illness.

The model of physician as fighter and victorious hero can be a two-edged sword. The doctor's personal engagement and consequent commitment to success can clearly be of benefit to the patient. At the same time, a misdirected desire to win may be at odds with the best interests of the patient. It can lead to overly aggressive and inappropriate interventions and a reluctance to change course since that may signal an ego-challenging retreat from the field of battle. This is especially evident in the surveys of health care delivery in the United States that reveal a preponderance of expenditures on acute care, especially in the last few months of life. A disease-oriented physician is less likely to engage the patient and family in such fateful discussions and decisions. Fighting can sometimes be desirable, but can be fraught with existential risks and emotional costs.

Patient versus Disease

A common variant of military metaphors in the discourse of medicine posits the patient as protagonist, engaged in battle and in a fight for his life with the enemy, disease. The patient gains direct agency in this formulation in contrast to the passive role in the first model we explored. The disease is still a reified entity, a thing, and the mission remains one of extirpation or destruction of the enemy. The patient continues to be regarded as containing or bearing a disease or morbid entity and removal constitutes cure. However, the patient is the macho agent and thereby acquires both a mode and sense of control and strategic power. The relationship of patient to physician is closer to that of an alliance and requires a particular sensibility on the part of the doctor, who must decipher the attitude of the person and adapt the mode of practice to accommodate the individual who is the patient. Some persons, often those with a military background, an abiding interest in sports, or whose career and life experience are rooted in making decisions and taking charge, may choose such an approach when they become patients. The metaphors by which they have lived prior to illness may be those of fighting and winning and these are then carried along into the "kingdom of the ill."

The physicians who work with such patients must learn to be more consultative and provide options and choices. They are careful to relinquish a degree of authority and autonomy and offer more advice and strategic directions. While both physician and patient remain engaged in the battle, power is now shared and distributed, in some instances involving members of the patient's family. There is a risk that certain physicians may choose to step back from the fray and perhaps become less engaged with a lesser commitment, not necessarily to the patient, but to the war against disease. After all, shared authority also entails shared responsibility that no longer rests solely with the doctor. Should that withdrawal continue, the patient may end up rather isolated and lonely.

A patient who wishes to be the protagonist may, in the course of illness, learn that the role may be valuable, but only when things are going well. When the battle is being won and the patient senses victory, this particular model may be empowering and helpful. However, the emotional landscape may change dramatically when problems and complications arise. If responsibility for a poor outcome is attributed to the passive patient described in the model in which the physician is leader and protagonist, then the assignment of blame is all the more focused when the patient is the fighter. After all, the person who opts for control and adopts the stance of a fighter may become a loser, albeit heroic, in the face of defeat. In the case of the patient, the price of desiring agency is an acceptance of blame. This is all the more difficult in this particular framing since the role of patient-protagonist is chosen, and the responsibility is elected, rather than imposed.

A deeper dilemma lies at the heart of the patient-fighting-the-disease model. The prevalent Western cultural trope, or at least the American image, is that of a fighter, and fighting the good fight is touted as more important than winning. This framing both energizes the military metaphors of medicine and is, in turn, promulgated by them. This shared societal value may impose an imperative on the patient to be a fighter exemplified by such exhortations from family and friends to the newly diagnosed patient as "You can beat this disease!" "We're with you all the way!" and "Never give up!" Some patients see this as welcome support, but others are uncomfortable and experience this as an added burden from cheerleaders at what is construed as a gladiatorial arena. The social and familial expectation to fight overwhelms the patient's reluctance so that any misgivings are kept hidden from family members and the treating physician alike. In other words, some patients are reluctant to share concerns about overly aggressive interventions and their attendant side effects and feel compelled to go on wearing the mantle of the fighter to avoid disappointing others. Stories from autopathographies of patients suffering from malignant disease have even described a sense of cowardice or being viewed as wimpy.

Among the unintended consequences of the role of fighter is the demand to always present the face of optimism, despite side effects and setbacks. This follows the public examples of well-known politicians or media stars who are photographed entering or leaving treatment centers with a cheerful thumbs-up, flashing a smile for the paparazzi. Teddy Kennedy and John McCain come readily to mind as role models for other patients to emulate. This dilemma was showcased in a piece in the *New York Times*, entitled "When Thumbs Up is No Comfort,"[9] which cited a cancer center social worker: "But patients say, 'I have to be positive, I can't cry, I can't let myself fall apart.' And that is a burden." The article notes that patients "feel guilty for not being as upbeat as the celebrities appear, and angry that the gravity of the disease is being misrepresented. By being constantly reminded that they should keep their chin up, patients implicitly believe that emotional wobbliness will adversely affect their outcome." Thus, not only can some patients not conform to what is expected of them, they face the added fear that the failure may worsen their prognosis. A medical ethicist underlined the sense of loneliness and isolation experienced by some patients by noting, "We only hear about those who handle it well," and "As a society we value the stoic but we don't know what the stoicism hides."[10]

The imperative to fight, especially when imposed by physicians or family and friends, becomes a harsh responsibility that may result in a sense of shame when victory becomes impossible. Upset at having disappointed the backers in her corner, the weary fighter is ready to withdraw from the ring. Coupled with the fear of the unknowable and the anxiety of uncertainty, the attendant shame may lead to despair, depression, and isolation from the much-needed structures of caring and support.

Unlike the urging of military field commanders to fight with the prospect of great victory and success, exhortations to patients to fight are not accompanied by a promise to win or even an end to the conflict. To the patient, the battle is never-ending and, at times, seems fated to be lost. Even the victory of survivorship, as we have noted, feels partial and often brings a liminal state that is best forgotten.

Susan Sontag eloquently described the "conventions of concealments with cancer,"[11] a disease "felt to be obscene,"[12] that leads to "all this lying to and by cancer patients." Though less common today, physicians and family members concealed the diagnosis from the patient, who was, more often than not, keenly aware of the situation. The patient, in turn, wishing to protect family members from the dire news, hid the fear and confusion and chose to be a stalwart fighter. Sontag noted, "Having a tumor generally arouses some feelings of shame."[13] Thus, the already attendant secrecy concealed the shame beneath the stoic face and was further exacerbated by the ignominy of not battling sufficiently bravely with its consequence of defeat. The frequent result was a lonely patient, suffering in silence and isolation.

In sum, the patient as protagonist is offered the opportunity to fight, exert control, and perhaps express a premorbid personality preference and a desire to take charge. This stance remedies in part the passivity of the patient as battleground and, with the cooperation of a thoughtful and sensitive physician, can lead to an alliance that may alleviate the isolation of illness. There are, nonetheless, costs to be considered. The battle is not for the faint of heart and even brave survivors may continue to live with continuing fears of recurrence. The fatigue due to the disease and the side effects of treatments are compounded by the demands of making choices that require clarity of mind and decisiveness of temperament. Both may be lacking when complications and difficulties arise. Turns for the worse can entail the burdens of blame and shame and regret for irrevocable choices. The sense of loss can be aggravated by a splintering of the therapeutic alliance as the physician withdraws from the field, abandoning the patient to suffer alone.

Physician as Mercenary

A variant of the patient-protagonist fighting with disease casts the physician as a mercenary, rather than as an ally. After all, many wars, both historical and modern, are fought with the aid of hired fighters and the physician is similarly engaged by the patient as an expert in medical combat. This model is consonant with a framing of care in which the patient becomes well informed through the Internet and other sources of data and is an autonomous agent in self-directed medical care. One common example is a man with high PSA values and a prostate biopsy indicative of low-grade localized malignancy. Several reasonable treatment options are available, including watchful waiting, local radiation, and radical prostatectomy. An individual in this situation, often educated and with the resources to seek information and visit many treatment centers, may choose to make the selection he feels appropriate and then seek a urologist who is willing to provide the desired care and intervention. While models of physicians who functioned as medical servants to the wealthy and relied on them for their livelihoods were commonplace in eighteenth-century England and elsewhere, this mode disappeared with the professionalization of doctoring. However, the advent of the Internet and highly specialized treatment centers advertising their offerings, coupled with the commercialization and corporatization of medicine, have reinvigorated this model of patient autonomy, with the physician as mercenary—all rather compatible with the metaphor of war.

The benefits and risks for the patient who opts for this particular approach are similar to those cited previously but are, in some sense, exaggerated. The doctor fights on behalf of patient as a hired gun and can provide advice as the patient chooses. However, professional input may be more constrained, the doctor may be less engaged in the course of illness, and the medical contribution more episodic in form. This mode places the individual person in the role of pilot and strategist. The patient is clearly in control and engaged and, with success, may be content with good health outcomes and take pride in making good decisions. The physician is shielded from major responsibility and has no incentive to provide superfluous interventions. At the same time, the medical mercenary can more readily withdraw once the contract has been executed. With poor outcomes, however, the patient is saddled with full responsibility and may come to face a lonely end on the field of battle with its sad echo, "It was your choice."

Commonly, patient autonomy requires that the health care provider avoid making decisions for the patient, and its advent is purported to signal a "more enlightened era of care."[14] This approach, often termed *patient-directed care*, may be beneficial for self-selected patients, but must not be imposed. At the same time, this choice can represent a challenge to older physicians who recall a traditional model of medicine in which doctors expected their advice to be heeded. Mitigating the risks for both parties requires a thoughtful, sensitive, and sensible clinician who accepts the obligation to shape an individualized and customized relationship responsive to the idiosyncrasies of each and every patient.

Disease as the Enemy of Society

This mode moves from an individual to a collective protagonist in which an entire nation, group, or indeed, the world, is threatened by disease. The latter remains reified and sometimes anthropomorphized as evil or monstrous and represents an abstracted, aggregated entity. Disease looms even larger in the plural, referring to countless numbers of cases. The words and images of a disseminated adversary are often used to describe sudden disruptive epidemics such as Ebola virus or influenza or chronic, recurrent diseases such as multidrug-resistant tuberculosis. The latter has been referred to as the white plague in echo of the medieval Black Death due to bubonic or pneumonic plague. These are no longer simply personal threats but societal adversaries, a view shared by all, whether healthy or ill, and demand organized, collective measures and responses. This is the battle of the experts in public health and epidemiology that tends to garner public interest through dramatic headlines in the media with its banners of breaking news, much like the announcements of the outbreak of war. While the discourse of battle was commonly used to refer to externally acquired infectious agents such as bacteria, viruses, and parasites, the metaphor later extended to internal pathological lesions and disruptions. In the former instance, we witnessed the presidential war on polio, in the latter, on cancer. Further afield, the military trope was marshalled to battle other societal ills, such as poverty and opioid addiction, and more recently has been brought to bear on diverse social threats. Climate change, as new-found enemy, engages warriors with the pithy slogan, "Your planet needs you—unite to combat climate change."

The public images of disease, even as they have varied over time, are shaped by the language of warfare, battles, and perfidious invasions. The early link between cancer and the image of a crab was morphological, from Galen's description of a tumor with "a shape and form similar to a crab, and ... veins, like its legs, extending from both sides." Very soon, however, the attribution became based on behavior, with the creeping growth and invasiveness of tumors likened to the slow but inexorable motions of the crustacean. The supposedly insidious and subclinical nature of cancer, unlike infections with their fevers and chaotic pathophysiology, brought to mind a Trojan horse attack on an unwary city. As actual warfare changed, the model of cancer became that of an imperialist disease that spreads beyond its normal tissue boundaries by invasion and metastatic spread to establish foreign outposts and eventually conquer the body. The realization that certain illnesses were contagious pointed to other sources of disease, yet still insidious and creeping. Thus, fourteenth-century Italian yielded "influenza and malaria" and Greek provided "miasmas," all evil emanations from swamplands and noxious vapors. The increasing understanding of the spread of pestilence and epidemics via animals and human contact led from vapors to the sanitation movements and the early organization of public health, paralleled by the extraordinary advances in bacteriology of the late nineteenth century. Early knowledge of the immune defenses soon followed, and the notion of an ongoing war between microbes and the forces of bodily resistance became the dominant construct of disease for the twentieth century. In contemporary models for the new century, the war against infections has escalated with the discovery of many organisms resistant to multiple antibiotics, outbreaks of novel viruses, global pandemics, and the recrudescence of measles as a result of lax policies on and misunderstandings of vaccinations. In the field of malignancy, novel drugs to unleash the power of the immune system in fighting tumors has opened a new front in that war. A new trope for cancer has also appeared—namely, the metaphor of speed and a runaway train due to a genetic mutational loss of braking mechanisms in malignant cells that may enhance their invasion and spread. This new image may represent a postmodern fear of time warps amplifying older fears of invasions and dybbuks. The specific understanding and explanations of diseases at a given point in history depend on the predominant models of causality and pathogenesis—what remains more or less constant are the tropes of war and fighters. The military metaphor has proven resilient over many centuries of human language and understanding.

Patients and Doctors

While it may not be surprising to find diseases described as enemies, patients experience other adversaries during illness. A study of actual language use found important examples of violence metaphors in communications by patients and physicians in a setting of palliative care.[15] Many of these reflected the relationships we have described previously. Patients express a desire to fight but also articulate the sense of personal failure when there is no improvement: "I feel such a failure that I am not winning this battle," and "Do I wither and retreat from this weary battle?"[16] Some examples demonstrated the ill effects of aggressive treatments. Chemotherapy was "a big wave [that] hits you" and "they hit me with radiation for ten days."[17] In addition, the study unearthed battle metaphors used by patients to describe their striving to get access to novel treatments that also reflected "a suspicion that doctors ... do not always act in the patients' interests."[18] Patients, perhaps especially in hospice care, feel multiply embattled, by the disease, the treatments, the demands of families and friends, and even the professionals of the health care system.

Military Language in Wartime

Besides the who and the why of military metaphors in medical discourse, we may also ask, when? Health metaphors are more often used to describe the state of the economy in the winter months when instances and thoughts of illness are more prevalent and salient. There is also a temporal variation in the prevalence of war metaphors in describing diseases, though in this instance, over years rather than seasons. This pattern underscores the importance of context and the state of people's lives in the usage of various figurative tropes.

The Google Books database can be searched for the prevalence of words and phrases and their variation in occurrence over time. The search process also affords a comparison between usage in different corpora, in this instance, between American and British English. It comes as no surprise to find the word *war* increased in prevalence in writings appearing during World Wars I and II. A comparison of American and British English shows that the increase of usage of *war* is about the same in WWI but reveals a greater increase in British English during WWII. This may be a reflection of the greater impact of WWII on the daily lives of those living in the United Kingdom compared with America. There is also a time difference in the increases, with the American English data showing the increase delayed by about two years, perhaps reflecting the late entries of the United States into the two wars. A search for the phrase "war against disease" in the corpus of British English accessible via Google Books similarly reveals a several-fold increase of this military metaphor during the later years of both WWI and WWII. By contrast, however, the prevalence of this metaphoric usage of war is almost two-fold greater in American English during WWII than in British English. Thus, while the descriptive use of war seemed to be more salient at that time in the United Kingdom, the greater increase of metaphoric use (war against disease) in the United States may have been the result of the sociolinguistic appeal of the military metaphor in American culture. This speculation is supported by a parallel comparison of the phrases "war against tuberculosis" and "war on tuberculosis" that are readily identified in the American English corpus—yet, the Google Book search process fails to identify such usage in the British English corpus.

Thus, salience in general and metaphoric salience in particular rest both on the words in circulation at a given period and the social and cultural forces that shape figurative language. In a sense, linguistic relativity reveals differences not only between discrete languages but also among local usages and linguistic varieties. A particular language variant provides an inflected view of the world that one can refer to as culture. In turn, the cultural salience and choice of specific figurative tropes shape the language that evolves and is articulated. These findings underscore once again the intimate nexus among culture, language, figurative tropes, and our behaviors and beliefs.

5

Sources of the Military Metaphors of Medicine

[F]ever is not a disease, but a war against disease, undertaken by means of a powerful force possessed by spirit. No better remedy has been given living beings by nature in order that they may recover health, just as nothing better than war by means of which states under attack ... may regain their peaceful condition.

—Thomas Campanella, 1635

We use war metaphors to describe and understand disease, and they shape how we treat the illnesses that are part of the human condition. Indeed, war metaphors are engrained in our language and thoughts, which has, not surprisingly, led many scholars to wonder how these tropes became part of our daily discourse and to speculate on their origins. The ubiquity of these metaphors points to sources with common biological origins or those with great cultural power. Since many of our long-standing concepts of illness spring from well-known infections such as the plague, cholera, influenza, and polio, it is reasonable to search for the formulation of the goal of medicine as the conquest of disease in the responses to devastating contagious illnesses.

Pasteur's Germ Theory[1]

The adversarial nature of the relationship between the person and the body on the one hand, and the disease on the other, was underscored in the late nineteenth century by the discovery of bacteria as the causal agents of human infections. The descriptions of cellular and humoral immunity and the development of antitoxins and vaccines provided a blueprint for a war between the newly discovered agents of causality and the bodily mechanisms of resistance and defense. The battle against germs was a natural outcome of the dominance of acute, contagious and epidemic diseases in human history, coupled with the idea that illnesses are caused by the invasion into the body (and mind) of exogenous foreign elements. Scholars reasonably concluded that the origins and popularity of the military metaphors in medicine can be traced to Pasteur's germ theory of disease and the subsequent scientific and cultural power of that model.[1]

In *Illness as Metaphor* Susan Sontag writes, "The military metaphor in medicine first came into wide use in the 1880s, with the identification of bacteria as agents of disease"[2] noting the capacity of microbes to "invade" or "infiltrate," and making the connection to Robert Koch, who, in 1882, identified the bacterial causative agent of tuberculosis. In the rhetorical instance of cancer, Sontag emphasizes that the war metaphor has taken on "a striking literalness and authority"[3] and that the disease itself has become the enemy against which society wages war. In this framing, the metaphoric language of war describes both the disease as invasive and imperialist, and the treatments designed to eradicate and eliminate, which are aggressive in both their intents and side effects. The recent advent of novel agents that alleviate or lift the blockade of the immune system, thereby unleashing lymphocytes to destroy tumor cells, has brought the immune system into the fray.

In *The Scientific Voice*, dedicated to the discourses of and about science, Scott Montgomery provides a detailed analysis of military tropes in the era of Pasteur. He, too, traces the origins of the war metaphor to the discovery of bacterial causes of infectious diseases, describes this trope as the "reigning image system for all disease in Western culture"[4] and chooses the term "biomilitarism[5]" for this conceptual framework.

Earlier Sources

The notions of medicine as a battle and disease as an adversary were already apparent in the early to mid-nineteenth century, well before the identification of bacteria as agents of causality. For example, the German physician Carl Heinrich Schultz published an opus on pathology in 1844-45 and used the terms *Krankheitskampf* (fight against disease) and *Wehrprozess* (military process) to describe an elaborate schema of the organism—the human body—engaged in a life-and-death battle, and postulated three reactions of the body to the pathological matter.[6] First, eliminating the disease by expulsion, for example, vomiting or coughing; second, assimilating the causal force, rendering it harmless; and third, a defensive stance manifesting as inflammation and fever. This sophisticated, rather prescient construct of a military framing of pathology did not depend on notions of bacterial agents as the target of the battle. In this naturalist framework, the disease remains the enemy and the protagonist is the body itself in a defensive posture, providing the second of the two major adversarial configurations that are evident both historically and currently. The first is the battle of medicine and doctors against disease, and the second arrangement posits the body or nature as the protagonist. In both instances, the agency of the patient as person is absent or submerged.

Some contemporaries of Schultz decried what they considered a fanciful idea of war and battles and insisted on an empirical and non-romanticized viewpoint. Nonetheless, in 1847, the pathologist Rudolf Virchow, who wrote in support of a rationalist position, found himself using the same metaphoric language as Schultz. To quote Virchow, "We no longer regard the pus corpuscles as gendarmes ordered by the police state to escort over the border some foreigner or other who is not provided with a passport."[7] Thus, even Virchow's denial of the metaphoric stance was stated in strong imaginative language, though he may have intended to deride his contemporaries. A number of years later, the war metaphor is employed by the same Virchow when he applauds Ilya Metchnikoff's work on inflammation—the title of the laudatory review is "The Battle of Cells and Bacteria."[8] By 1901, Metchnikoff published his important pioneering work on cellular immunology, *Immunity in Infectious Diseases*[9] that develops the idea of a full-fledged biological system of defense against parasites. One may argue that in so doing Metchnikoff concretized the metaphor of war as a biological reality of phagocytes defending the body against foreign invaders. Thus, Schultz's figurative descriptions foretold the empirical findings of Metchnikoff, who continued to use the same figurative language to elaborate and explicate his emerging theories. For, after all, scientific theories are themselves metaphoric images of nature.

The military metaphor used in the mid-nineteenth century to describe various pathological processes provided a discourse to Pasteur and others, who, several decades later, used the notion of entry to describe exogenous organisms necessary for the production of wine and cheese by fermentation. Moreover, the invasion of such cultures of bread, wine, or cheese by unwanted bacteria or fungi led to the diseases of such products. The unrest in Europe that culminated in the Franco-Prussian war of 1870 may have enhanced the currency of war-like thoughts and language in the two countries that were home to exciting research in bacteriology and immunology. It was but a short step to consider bacteria as the shock troops of the enemy, disease. Conversely, Virchow, with his strong sense of social justice and societal improvement, used his newly found knowledge of cellular defense mechanisms and bacteriology to metaphorically characterize the contemporary social unrest and turmoil by describing the "Police-Organism" that uses an "imprisoning wall" of "scar tissue" to enclose "foreigners."[10] Thus, the biological body is the source, and societal exclusion is the target of the trope. At the same time, the prevailing military discourses, both metaphoric and descriptive, also set the stage for understanding the novel anti-toxins and phagocytes as members of the defense mechanisms of both humoral and cellular immunity that were elaborated in the late nineteenth and early twentieth centuries. The use of adversarial framings by the pioneers of immunology stimulated the efflorescence of the war metaphors in medicine that remain evident in both technical and informal discourses. In his 1914 address to the Tuberculosis Association, Sir William Osler encouraged his colleagues in public health by stating, "We have tracked the enemy, and know his very stronghold, and we know his three allies—poverty, bad housing, and drink. But though the ravages have been reduced it remains the most powerful among man's innumerable enemies. Before us is a long, slow, hundred years' war."[11] A similarly poetic description of the world of public health and medicine was composed by the American microbiologist Hans Zinsser, in 1935: "Infectious disease is one of the few genuine adventures left in the world. The dragons are all dead, and the lance grows rusty in the chimney corner.... About the only sporting proposition that remains unimpaired ... is the war against these ferocious little fellow creatures which lurk in the dark corners and stalk us in the bodies of rats, mice and all kinds of domestic animals; which fly and crawl with the insects, and waylay us in our food and drink and even in our love."[12] These constructs of surveillance, eradication, fine-grained distinctions between self and other, and defense and resistance remain the prevalent imagery for immunology to the present and have gained an added boost of energy with the advent of therapies for cancer that unblock killer T-lymphocytes and unleash them to destroy tumors.

Quotidian Discourse

Just as the military metaphor was evident in medical writings prior to Pasteur's publications, it also appeared in ordinary journals before bacterial infections were identified. A *New York Times* editorialist of April 7, 1860, writes of the "Samaritan profession whose pleasure it is to battle with disease and suffering in every conceivable form"[13]; on June 17, 1861, an editorial notes that "disease is the enemy by far the most to be dreaded"[14]; and on March 23, 1864, a letter describes a ship's physician who had "exhausted all the means in his power to combat the disease."[15] Across the Atlantic, the *Lloyd's Weekly London Newspaper* of February 27, 1848, includes a report entitled "The War Against Disease and Death,"[16] and the phrase, "war against contagion, disease and death"[17] appears in the *Aris's Birmingham Gazette* of July 17, 1848.

Medical Luminaries

The finding that war metaphors for medicine, disease, and the body date back to the mid-nineteenth century shifts the search for the origin story toward earlier sources, namely, the writings of medical luminaries of the sixteenth and seventeenth centuries in Europe, more particularly, England, Holland, and France. Thomas Sydenham, a founder of clinical medicine and bedside observation was known as the English Hippocrates who classified diseases into specific categories to permit accurate diagnoses. This form of taxonomy and the language Sydenham used to describe diseases reflected a shift from disease as an imbalance of humors to disease as a reified entity, a thing. This novel understanding of disease stemmed from the ideas promulgated by two philosophers of the mid-sixteenth and early seventeenth centuries, Paracelsus and von Helmont, who disagreed with the ancient notion that each person's disease was unique and due to an excess or deficiency of humors within. Von Helmont stated that diseases are "defects ... from an external Cause" and the result of "strange guests received within."[18] The earlier work by Paracelsus described both the new nature of disease and the need for battle, "when a disease is in the body, all the healthy organs of the body have to fight against it."[19] Ontologizing diseases transformed them from processes into objects, thus making them susceptible to elimination or extirpation. In that sense, this was a necessary step to viewing diseases as enemies to be conquered. Sydenham wrote of "ejecting the morbifick Matter" and cure entailed "expelling the Disease," thus "vanquishing the Intestinal Enemy."[20] He opined that the prevention of evacuation would lead to the destruction of the patient by "an Intestine War, his Enemy being kept in his bowels." This accomplished clinician understood fever and crises to be signs of the battles raging within the body and described a "destructive Troop of Diseases" which "wages War with Mankind every day.[21]" His Dutch colleague Herman Boerhaave introduced bedside teaching of medical students and envisaged the body as a mechanical entity. However, he, too, wrote of a cancerous growth as "the Evil" that must be removed and that "to heal therefore is to take away a disease from the Body."[22] French physician Pierre Brissot noted in 1522 that when "foreign substances" are being expelled from the body, "auxiliary troops" are sent "to beat down the common enemy"[23] (translation from Rather). These three pioneer physicians demonstrated in their writings an understanding of disease as an object and one that needs to be eliminated from the body and defeated in order to effect healing. Hence, the war metaphor anticipated, and may have provided the linguistic groundwork for, germ theory and the field of immunology that developed more than two centuries later.

Bellum contra Morbum

The earliest extant source that deploys fully developed imagery of a battle against disease within the body is the work of a seventeenth-century Dominican friar, Thomas Campanella. He lived in Italy and France and was a well-known philosopher and astrologer who produced a seven-volume opus dedicated to medicine. Published in 1635, it appears to have been written between 1610 and 1613, and the last of the seven volumes is dedicated to a disquisition on fever. He disagreed with the notions current in his time and stated that "fever is not a disease, but a war against disease [*febrem non esse morbum, sed bellum contra morbum*]."[24] Historians have noted that the catchphrase, *bellum contra morbum*, posits the idea that fever is the external evidence of a war being fought within the body that can "conquer and eject." The essence of fever is "expelling some significant evil." In his treatise, Campanella also refers to Galen's very rare use of the war metaphor by noting that Galen taught that fever is a sign of nature "desiring to do battle"[25] and is a "remedy against evils." A similar perspective was offered by another Italian astrologer, Peter of Abano, who lived three centuries earlier. He was also a physician and professor of medicine who studied the medical and philosophical treatises of Islamic scholars, and compared the "war between the body and the morbific matter ... to dueling boxers."[26]

The explicit linkage of source and target domains was evident in both Campanella and Galen, albeit in different directions. The former noted that just as metaphoric battles made evident by fever can result in recuperation, "nothing better than war has been found by means of which states under attack … may regain their peaceful condition."[27] Galen compared "discord within political states to disease." Both commentators, Campanella the philosopher and Galen the physician, explored the power of metaphors and their extensions to both understand the nature of fever and disease and to shed light on politics and nation-states via linguistic allusions and cognitive connections.

The Moral Nature of Disease

Physicians and philosophers of the sixteenth and seventeenth centuries provide early evidence of war metaphors with battles against disease and the linkage between expulsion and healing. These early forerunners of modernity and rationalism also provide the linguistic traces of the understandings of disease they carried forward from earlier medieval framings. Paracelsus noted that diseases "arise like Lucifer in the heavens out of their own upstart pride."[28] He then draws an explicit parallel between the fight against disease and its evil nature: "In the same way, you can see how the soul must struggle against the devil with all of its powers."[29] Paracelsus declared that "human passion—wanton lust, volition, fury" is "directly convertible into a disease-body."[30] Von Helmont elaborated this connection by adding a nuance to the comparison between disease and sin. Disease, according to von Helmont, is an "evil in respect of Life" and it "arose from Sin."[31] Yet it differs in that sin arises from a deficiency, presumably moral, whereas disease requires an efficient cause. This illustrates the transition between the medieval notion of disease as a consequence of sinfulness and the later construct of a reified entity that is "actual and real." More generally, von Helmont thought that "disease broke over man after the Fall when he laid himself open to foreign seeds and disease."[32]

Sydenham was keen to "bridle the fury of the disease" by evacuating what he described as the "peccant Humour."[33] The archaic word, *peccant*, has multiple meanings, including an adjective for something that is diseased and a thing that is sinful. Peccant as a noun refers to a sinner, and is derived from the Latin, *peccare*, meaning "to sin." This dual use reflects the relatedness of disease and sin in English and describes the entities that Sydenham wished to conquer and eliminate—the disease by certain medications and the sin by moral interventions. Perhaps they were functionally linked! Similarly, Boerhaave described a hard growth as a scirrhus, which, if disturbed becomes a cancer that reacts by "shooting its malignant Roots everywhere deep into the adjacent Muscles and Vessels."[34] He recommended "the keeping of the Evil dormant and quiet." Cancer was figuratively, yet explicitly, linked to sinfulness: Francis Bacon wrote in 1597 that "Enuie … is the canker of Honour,"[35] and related citations from the OED refer to "that pestylent and most infectuous canker, ydlenes" (1564),[36] and "Sloth is a Cancer, eating up that Time Princes should cultivate for Things sublime" (1711).[37]

An elaborate example of the understanding of disease and its origins is available in a treatise on syphilis, published in 1496 by the German astrologer Joseph Grünpeck von Burckhausen. *A Neat Treatise on the Origin of the French Evil,* written at a time when syphilis was rampant in Europe, discussed the astrological conditions conducive to the outbreaks of this disease and linked its etiology to divine sources. Grünpeck wrote that "new diseases" are "the arrows of the gods, with which wickedness becomes cleansed and chastised, and badness is driven out."[38] He then cites a series of biblical sources to conclude that sickness is "a plague sent by God to humans … as a punishment to mortals on account of sin."[39] This perspective is articulated in a sermon by the poet John Donne, likewise citing a biblical source to conclude that "the first cause of death, and sickness, and all infirmities upon mankind in general, was sin."[40]

The Puritan reformation in seventeenth-century England showcased the connections between disease and sin, body and soul, and physicians and ministers. While Protestant theology rejected saintly miracles and the cure of illness by priestly intervention, it nonetheless underscored the phenomena of death and disease as the consequences of sinfulness. "Sickness comes usually and ordinarily from sin"[41] wrote the great Puritan theologian, William Perkins. Life was understood in spiritual terms and divine influence was clear and quotidian. The great plagues of London were due to the Lord's wrath evoked by human sinfulness and the three arrows of retribution—the sword, famine, and disease. Body and soul were interconnected—"the body was the instrument of the soul"[42]—a diseased body impaired the expression of the soul. Conversely, a physician could not heal a body in the face of a sinful soul. Repentance was an a priori requisite to curing. This conjoint nature of the person implied a collegial partnership between physician and minister—the former dealing with the body, the latter with the soul. The need for intervention by both and the interfaced roles are reminiscent of an older tradition of physicians as priests of the temple of Asklepios and the theological concept of Christ as Physician. This dual nature of the healing/pastoral professions underscored the connections of disease and sin not only in the sense of causality but also with regard to therapeutics and healing.

This relationship is also evident in the ready interchange of metaphors between the two traditions. To cite Perkins, "the curing of the disease fitly resembleth the curing of sin"[43] and, conversely, disease could be purged when the repentant patient's sins had been purged. The language of medicine, of cures, could be readily applied to the alleviation of sinfulness, and the language of ritual and of the Bible, that of purgations, was used to describe elimination of body contents, including "morbifick matter." The OED traces both meanings of purgation, the moral and the physical, to the fourteenth century—and purgatory is itself a venue of spiritual cleansing and purification. Perkins also offered a comment that may hearten our contemporary doctors of the soul, namely, psychiatrists, as follows: "he made confession of them [his sins] unto God, and thereupon obtained his pardon, and was healed."[44]

Disease and the Search for Meaning

Humans need to make sense of the phenomena of the worlds we inhabit—we discern patterns in nature and tell stories of causality that help us understand the past and anticipate the future. We need to diminish uncertainty and are not comfortable with randomness and chance. In a word, we seek to ascribe meanings to our experiences, not least among them, disease and illness. By the late Middle Ages in Europe, that is, early in the fourteenth century and increasingly by the mid-seventeenth century, disease became entwined and understood in a moral universe. As the notion of disease shifted from imbalances of natural forces to a reified entity, it became tainted with images of evil and malignity, and in moral terms, disease was the outcome of sinfulness and emblematic of punishment for transgressions. These emerging frameworks caused disease to become synonymous with sins and, thus, the target of a moral fight intended to regain both purity and health.

This picture is quite different from the understanding of disease in ancient Greece. Vivian Nutton, a scholar of ancient medicine, describes "the general absence of any linkage between disease and sin."[45] At sacred temples "the patient made a bargain for the future, not a repentance for the past." While there was belief in the supernatural as explanatory mechanism, illness was not viewed as punishment for sins. As Nutton notes, "If, as in the famous plague that begins Homer's *Iliad*, disease was the result of divine wrath, its cause was more a ritual offence against the god than any moral transgression."[46] Even in instances of "illness as a divine punishment ... [it was] for a specific cult offence, not a moral failing." The Greek and Roman systems of beliefs did not encompass "the crowds of demons which infested the world of the Bible" nor "the malignant demons ... of the New Testament."[47] Finally, Nutton describes a crucial feature that distinguishes ancient beliefs from Judeo-Christian frameworks, as follows: "Individual illness is less caught up in the eternal struggle between the mysterious forces of good and evil; bodily infirmity is explicable on physical, not moral grounds."[48] Thus, a critical inflection point in the meaning of illness and disease and their place in a moral universe is the transition between ancient Greek and Roman medicine and the advent of early Christianity with its radically different theological framework.

The *Psychomachia*

The framing of disease in moral terms provides a mechanism of causation and, thereby, an explanation for the advent of puzzling and strange illnesses that appear to strike randomly and yet selectively. If the causal agents are simply parts of nature, then if one person is stricken down with the plague, then all should become so afflicted. Yet, it was clear to ancient and medieval observers that some were spared while others perished. However, if diseases are either retributions for prior sins or, at the least, admonitory lessons to avert future immorality, then, in addition to natural causes, one must consider features of the moral life and constitution of the persons so stricken or spared.

A broad canvas that offers a backdrop for these notions was provided by early Christian writers and scholars whose ideas prefigured and foreshadowed the later theological concepts promulgated by Puritans and other early modern movements. Perhaps the premier example is the *Psychomachia*, an extended poem composed early in the fifth century AD by the late-ancient Roman-Christian, Aurelius Prudentius. In this work, whose title is often translated as *Battle of the Soul*, the poet describes the epic battles between good and evil to gain dominance over the soul of a person. The armies deployed in this sweeping allegory are those of the virtues of faith in a holy war with the vices of idolatry. Allegories are characterized by double meanings with a written text or narrative intending a hidden message, often a moral theme emerging from a battle or conflict. The dramatis personae in allegories are often personified abstractions with agency. In this particular early example we meet Hope, Sobriety, Chastity, and Humility, fighting and defeating Pride, Wrath, Lust, and Avarice. For example, Chastity, the virgin queen, defends herself against Lust, her arch-enemy from Sodom—and emerges triumphant! On one level, the poem is in the style of heroic Greek war stories. At the same time, the underlying narrative is one of early embattled Christians reaching out to convince their pagan countrymen to convert to the newly emerging faith. On an individual level, the holy war between good and evil is an internal battle of ideas between a person's good and evil dispositions, each seeking domination of the soul. These two contrasting human attributes are traced biblically to the Fall of Man that, in Christian theology, led to the existence of evil and sins in the world of humans. While the Judaic tradition does not speak of the biblical Fall, it nonetheless describes the *yetzer hatov*[49] and the *yetzer hara*, the good and evil inclinations, respectively.

The allegorical symbolic power struggles between good and evil in apocalyptic abstractions become for each individual a fight between dueling inclinations or between the spirit of virtue and the self of vice. In psychoanalytic terms, we speak of the superego and the id that vie for control of personality. It may seem paradoxical that virtue engages in battles—yet, the Christian notion of virtue as moral excellence is preceded linguistically by an older idea of virtue as energy, fortitude or valor. Thus, virtue needs strength to conquer vice. By contrast, a weak, that is, non-virtuous, disposition is prone to sinfulness that can bring retributive disease in its wake. A magisterial work on allegory by Angus Fletcher notes that "sin came naturally to be identified with plague, since plague was a reality in Europe well on into the eighteenth century."[50] In its allegorical framing, Disease can be averted by resisting Sin that requires stalwart spiritual battle; "the disease is the product of the breath (*miasma*) of Satan ... and the Black Plague itself ... was an effluence of evil spirits floating through the air."[51] In short, once Disease becomes seen as evil, malign, and identified with sin, then it, too, must be fought by the body, just as Virtue battles Vice. Over the span of modernity, the *Psychomachia* has been updated from good versus evil to nature versus disease to person (or physician) versus disease.

Dirt, Disease, and Sins

The historian Owsei Temkin has pointed out that the "Latin *infectio* means ... staining or dyeing ... so that something ... becomes tainted, spoiled or corrupted,"[52] and it is analogous to the Greek *miasma* or pollution. Thus, plague shifted in causality from an impurity in the soul to a pollutant in the air to a bacterium in the blood—in all instances, entities that must be fought. What connects these three forms of corruption, namely, of the soul, the air, and the blood by sins, pollutants, and bacteria? These are all forms of "dangerous contagion" that threaten established order, social classifications, and well-being. Anthropologist Mary Douglas described dirt as that which "offends against order,"[53] and defilement is disorder that transgresses boundaries. To protect against such forces that present dangers to societies, we construct codes and guidelines to regulate and control human behaviors to avert or mitigate the threats to hygiene and civility. A culture chooses appropriate means to "confront events which seem to defy its assumptions."[54] Moral codes are constructed as constant reminders of the allegorical battle between good and evil and designed to motivate behaviors that eschew sins and transgressions. In the Judeo-Christian tradition, "holiness and impurity are at opposite poles"[55] and attaining the necessary degree of spiritual hygiene is the objective of an array of guides to healthy living. The recognition of pollutants in the air, miasmas and ghostly fogs, or, in modern understandings, lead-contaminated water and sulfurous smogs led to epidemic surveillance and laws to protect the public health. Finally, bacteria may be associated with dirt and pollution, both figuratively and literally. They are traditionally, perhaps erroneously, linked to excrement, death, and sites of filth and neglect. Bacteria are both contagious and transgressive by crossing boundaries into the human body and are offensive by disrupting the established order of health and homeostasis. Thus, they threaten individual hygiene and the good order of well-being. There is a continuity between the sacred and the secular in the need for the societal regulation of human affairs that may undermine the commonweal and endanger the persons who constitute society. This is evident in language—defilement and contamination describe sins and parasites while purgation and cleansing are means of purifying bodies and souls. While our secular society no longer refers to sins or perhaps even moral codes as wellsprings for behavior, the ancient, centuries-old association between bacteria and defilement continues as a deeply rooted cultural trope. That may explain our astonishment at the discovery of the microbiome and the realization that beneficial bacteria are ubiquitous and necessary for human health and survival.

Allegories construct broad conceptual frameworks, provide metaphysical causal explanations, and have immense, long-lasting, symbolic and narrative power. They link macrocosmic forces with the microcosms of daily existence and help us make sense of why things happen as they do. A predominant allegorical form is that of an epic battle of mythic proportions over great spans of time. It is this formulation viewed in historical evolution that may help us trace the genealogy of the war-like linguistic tropes so common in medicine (please see Table 5.1, Tropes of War).

The headwaters for this flow of ideas are in the biblical story in Genesis of the Fall and the consequential introduction of evil into the cosmic narrative. While different traditions have important variations, the Christian interpretation provides, on a grand sweep, the fateful framework of original sin introduced into a pristine and pure world. On a macrocosmic, perhaps heavenly scale, an agent of the Divine strives to protect humankind from the blandishments of Satan. On an earthly, microcosmic level, each individual soul is the object of the opposing forces of Good and Evil delineated in *The Psychomachia,* engaged in a never-ending fight that entails constant vigilance. The external manifestations of this inner turmoil are the personal behaviors reflecting the waxing and waning influences of Virtue and Sin, whose foot soldiers are on daily deployment. Many examples can be adduced to illustrate the numerous variants of this allegorical construct in Western literature and history. The Crusades of the Middle Ages to liberate the Holy City of Jerusalem from non-Christian occupiers were carried out by knights known as *milites Christi* (soldiers of Christ) engaged in a battle to rid the City of the occupying invaders and restore it to its heavenly purity. Indeed, the theme of defilement was evident in Crusader documents and religious tracts. While this is not a medical or biological example, it underscores the pervasive nature of this particular allegory, in particular in instances where purity and wholeness are germane.

The defended city of the Crusades maps quite readily onto the human body, often described figuratively as a holy stronghold. It is the field of play of defense mechanisms of the immune and other protective systems that resist or destroy invading germs. The language of war and contending forces now seems quite natural to us and many of the metaphors have become burnished by usage and somewhat literalized. That brings us to our familiar metaphor of the patient as passive battleground on which the heroic physician engages with the arch-enemy, disease. These instances are not intended to describe a strict chronology. Rather, they show how the allegory of Good and Evil evolves over time, ramifies into overlapping networks of meaning,

Table 5.1 Tropes of War

Positive Force	Battleground	Opposing Force
Divine agent	Humankind	Satan
Good	Soul	Evil
Virtue	Person	Sin
Knight	City	Invader
Defenses	Body	Germs
Doctor	Patient	Disease

and is in turn reshaped by the particular contexts—linguistic, social, and cultural—of the given moment in history. The basic idea, however, remains robust and influential throughout.

Cultural Change and Stability

How does an idea retain an enduring influence over the span of a millennium and more? In his 1935 book, *The Heavenly City of the Eighteenth-Century Philosophers*, American historian Carl Becker traced the evolution of the concept of a Heavenly City from its medieval sources to a new framing by the rationalist philosophers of the eighteenth century, particularly in revolutionary France. He wrote that "the Heavenly City thus shifted to earthly foundations"[56] and that the ancient transcendent idea was altered but did not disappear—it took on new forms and descriptors. The *philosophes* remained in debt to medieval thought and the Revolution retained a "religious character" and a grand narrative of redemption. The Enlightenment was, in his view, not a sharp break with the past but rather a reshaped narrative with enduring themes. Becker wrote of "climates of opinion" that change with time and whose traces are evident in language and tropes characteristic of the time. Thus, words with currency in the thirteenth century were "God, sin, grace, salvation, and heaven,"[57] all reflective of the Fall and the dominant medieval theology. In its place, the thinkers of the Enlightenment put their faith in reason, empiricism, and skepticism. Yet, these philosophers were not cold-blooded, indifferent rationalists but rather enthusiasts with passion for a "New Religion of Humanity." A belief in the Divine was supplanted by doctrine based on Nature. The words of the eighteenth century, wrote Becker, were "nature, natural law, first cause, and reason."[58] A need to understand agency and a stance rooted in teleology was replaced by an interest in mechanisms—a shift from why to how.

And yet the loss of belief, faith, and awe and an accompanying disappearance of goodness, virtue, justice, and sentiment resulted in a need for a framework grounded in more than the coldness of pure reason. As Becker noted, "the soul that Cartesian logic had eliminated from the individual had to be rediscovered in humanity."[59] The new religion of a "deified nature"[60] sought the good life on earth, rather than in heaven, and the eighteenth-century philosophers spoke of the natural rights of man, the Great Book of Nature, and a Prime Mover. The mode of worship was a transcendental humanism and the object was the perfectibility of Man with his natural rights to justice and freedom. Morality returned through the back door with a focus on the amelioration of society and social movements to cope with the evident resistance of Evil to yield to Reason. The Heavenly City of medieval theology gave birth to an earthly Jerusalem, and the need of humans for drama led to an efflorescence of early nineteenth-century prophets for humanity with their own rituals and arcana. Thus, ancient allegories evolve and mutate but yet retain a core of beliefs reflected in language and behavior.

Two Evolving Strands

The evolution of military tropes over time points to two entwined strands. The post-lapsarian chronology traces back to the biblical narrative and the resultant psychomachia of the early Christians. These ideas give rise to the battle between good and evil that links the fight against sins and evil inclinations to latter-day models of the role of the physician (or patient) to wage war against disease. The second strand originates in the medieval ideas of fever as evidence of the internal battles of the body coping with afflictions and invasions of morbific matter. This naturalist explanation foreshadows the germ theory of Pasteur and the subsequent developments of immunology and the scientific understanding of defense mechanisms of the body. What interweaves the two threads are the metaphoric links of sins, defilement, and dirt to the medieval plagues and the concurrent understanding that such evils and epidemics are the results of transgressions and depravity. Even in the twentieth century, when the knowledge of infections, viruses, and bacteria are widespread, we continue to live with our ancient notions that certain diseases are dirty and somehow emanate from the dark side. Leprosy may be gone, but the stigma and taint remain.

6

Consequences of the Verbal Wars

Advice to a Bristol medical student in the late eighteenth century: "Give early Relief to your Patient and it will be a means of gaining his confidence and esteem, then attack the Disease more radically."[1]

—Mary Fissell

Our understanding of disease shapes the work of physicians, their relationships with patients, and the provision of care. The perception of disease as an object can be traced to Europe in the middle of last millennium, and the metaphors that resonate to this day stem from notions of causality that are older, yet again.

Disease and Diagnosis

Appreciating disease as a thing rather than a process implies that patients are carriers or containers that bring diseases to their physicians, saying, for example, "I think I had a cold and now I may have pneumonia." This statement may be accompanied by an admission of responsibility, as in, "I caught it while walking outdoors in the winter weather!" Possessing a disease suggests that it has an independent existence and can become the object of interest and the focus of attention for the clinician. Diagnosis is thereby transformed into a search for a lesion and its cause. Physicians have often been described as medical detectives embroiled in a who-done-it search for the culprit. The patient is the source of clues that point to lines of inquiry: for example, a child's skin rash may point to the causal virus harbored within. A particular skill at diagnosis has unfortunately become the prime index of a clinician's renown among patients and a spur to hero worship for medical students and residents. Acumen is the attribute that describes success at diagnostics, and such skills are celebrated in clinical-pathological conferences, or CPCs, that have appeared weekly for more than a century in the most widely read medical publication, the *New England Journal of Medicine*. The overweening importance of diagnosis is also mirrored by the fame of consultative centers to which patients may be referred when "no-one knows what's wrong."

Deciphering the cause of a patient's ailment is important to both patient and physician. For both, it represents the elimination of uncertainty and a welcome solution to a mystery. For patients, attaching a name to an illness has added value in reducing fear of the unknown, reflected in the aphorism naming is taming. Even when the diagnostic process uncovers a serious illness, a patient may feel relieved and even joyful at finally understanding what is wrong. This happy response may seem paradoxical—yet, a patient may not find comfort in being told by a physician that "Everything seems to be fine." Rather than a description of good health, it may actually mean, "I am unable to understand your illness." The patient whose symptoms and distress continue notwithstanding such reassurance may conclude that the physician is not able to determine the nature of the illness causing the patient's concern or, worse yet, is not fully engaged in the situation. Other equally unhappy possibilities are a rare and unusual illness. The unknown generates fear. More often, however, a patient in such circumstances feels neglected by a physician who may be embarrassed by a lack of a clear diagnosis and, in some instances, the sufferer may be told that there is nothing wrong or "it is all in your head." The patient feels diminished and may be regarded as uncooperative by the physician. In certain chronic illnesses, such seeming disregard may go on for months or years and motivate visits to multiple consultants seeking an answer—as well as respect. In such settings, the clarity of a definitive diagnosis, even if dire, represents a long-awaited validation of the patient as a truthful witness and, perhaps, a turning point in the clinical relationship and the process of care.

A diagnostic label is useful and important to patients, physicians, and epidemiologists and administrators for whom large databases and taxonomies are useful. However, both the reification of disease and the overweening emphasis on diagnosis entail untoward and perhaps harmful consequences. The traditional methods of classification of diagnosis relied heavily on pathological descriptions of the alterations in morphology of the affected tissues. These may include, for example, sites of inflammation, infections, aberrant growth of tumors, and structural or traumatic malformations. Thus, diseases are recognized through a microscope or imaging methods such as X-rays or computed tomography (CT) scans and manifest as physical realities. In many instances, the definitive diagnostic procedure is a tissue biopsy. This emphasis on the physically visible tends to undermine the validity for physicians, though not for patients, of illnesses that cannot be seen, including impairments of mental health, psychosomatic conditions, closed head injuries, and other forms of suffering and angst with impairments of function. Objectification of diseases has also led to a strong reliance on and attention to taxonomies of disease rather than classifications based on patients' loss of functional capacities and their impacts on daily living.

An interesting effect of the taxonomy of diseases as the guiding principle in medicine is described by Justin Mutter, a geriatrician and ethicist, in a paper on the "political economy of diagnosis."[2] He notes that health care for the elderly in the United States is supported by Medicare, whose payments are linked to specific diagnostic entities. Once reimbursement is tied to such classifications, care becomes "thoroughly reductionist," leading to care as a series of "fractured transactions" rather than "a unifying mission of well-being." This "biomedical atomization ... recasts human health as a mere sum of its parts."[3] He recommends a framework based on a regime of prognosis for the whole person with attention to functional improvements through modest, stepwise interventions, regardless of the specific disease label. Finally, Mutter notes that there is no disease classification for "frailty," yet that is the actual state of many who need care in the later years of life.

The magnification of the diagnostic gaze has focused attention to increasingly smaller fields of view and has enhanced the fine discriminations in the classification of certain diseases. Around 1800 and in the two decades that followed, physicians of the Paris School devised methods of examination of the exterior of the body that yielded information on the pathological changes within. Thus, Laennec's stethoscope and Corvisart's technique of percussion made accessible to the medical gaze evidence of a pneumonia or pleurisy in the chest. A century later, Röntgen's X-ray machine allowed physicians to peer inside the body, perhaps directly at the disease within, and garnered a Nobel Prize for the inventor. A century after that, a Nobel Prize was awarded for the design of the magnetic resonance imaging (MRI) technique to visualize diseases inside the body.

The reification of disease and its transformation into an object permitted the search for the seat of disease in the body, a phrase that stems from the Latin title of Giovanni Morgani's great work, *De Sedibus et Causis Morborum*. As a result, the attention of the physician is directed to the object of interest and away from its carrier or vessel, the patient. The body is a delivery package for the disease within and the signs and symptoms are labels and clues to the content. The evolution over a span of two centuries of techniques for the diagnostic search led to the stepwise narrowing of the field of interest with a reduction of focus along the pathway of reification so that a genetic disease may now be found in a misshapen molecule due to an error in DNA orthography. The patient's body, at first open to the medical gaze of the internist, became accessible to the radiologist, and is now wholly transparent to the modern imaging specialist. The aim of MRI is to visualize pure disease, unobstructed by the patient, and the person is a ghost on the computer screen. Recent technological advances have directed our interest to other kinds of diagnostic clues, namely alterations of molecules, biochemical pathways, and genetic mutations and other changes to the genome. Now, the body and patient have become superfluous to the molecular physician, who tracks the data from the gene sequencer. The patient is not simply open to the medical gaze but rendered completely irrelevant to it. Diagnosis remains a search for changes of structure, whether of whole organs, tissues, or molecules of DNA. The psyche, totally invisible and ephemeral from the perspective of imagers and the archeologists and pathologists of DNA, lies abandoned on the analyst's couch.

The reified disease, abstracted from the contexts of particular patients, is readily classified and understood as a pure form with clear diagnostic and taxonomic criteria. This framing satisfies the physician's desire for simple diagnostic clarity and the useful shorthand of a well-known label. A diagnosis can be free from the messy particularity of an individual patient and ignores those elements of the person that may not fit neatly into the chosen category. Of course, the patient knows only particularity and seeks attentiveness to all the details that make the person unique. Thus, the interests of the physician and patient, while they may not have diverged completely, are now distinguishable and not entirely congruent. "Disease entities have become indisputable social actors,[4]" is the apt description of the reification of disease and its diagnostic labels articulated by historian Charles Rosenberg in a paper entitled "The Tyranny of Diagnosis." The disease is the interlocutor for the physician and is the surrogate for the person who is ill and who is thus set aside as a matter of concern. The most significant result of this rearrangement is the shift of the medical gaze over a span of two centuries, from person, to patient, to organ, to lesion, and, finally, to the computer screen. To be clear, this is not evidence of uncaring or apathetic clinicians. It is rather the result of what Baziak and Dentan have termed "cultural and linguistic preconditioning."[5] Health professionals are embedded in a specific subculture and behave in accordance with the accumulated social norms and habits of the craft.

The framing of disease as specific entities has intensified with technological change and the hegemony of diagnosis. This understanding is deeply flawed and is unable to account for the complexity of diseases and the contingencies relevant to their actual etiologies and clinical courses. Infectious diseases are described as needing both seed and soil for their genesis. That is, bacteria alone do not cause disease—they require an appropriate environment for growth and the elaboration of their latent pathogenicity. In an apocryphal story, Max Joseph Pettenkofer, a skeptical colleague of Robert Koch, drank a broth containing the newly discovered Vibrio cholera and failed to develop the disease. This was an early and dramatic illustration of the well-known concepts of public health that diseases are multifactorial in their causality and many factors are necessary, some of them idiosyncratic to the individual patient, yet relevant to the course of illness.

Disease and Illness

The medical anthropologist Arthur Kleinman proposed the instructive distinction between disease and illness, noting that the former is the object of interest to the physician, while illness connotes the experience of the individual patient. The former is nomothetic; the latter, idiographic. Disease, as we have seen, is readily and, perhaps, necessarily abstracted, generalized, and objectified, whereas illness is inexorably unique, specific, and subjective. Illness has limited existence within the frame shaped by the military metaphors, especially with a medical protagonist and a passive patient. Disease evokes a diagnostic model that is agent-centered (who-done-it) while illness is patient-centered and demands engagement with messy details, particular concerns, and a sense of the patient's inner life. The concept of illness comprises all the factors and features that influence and shape the cause, course, management, and outcome of an illness. These include the person's prior experiences, purposes, goals, and desires. The full array of genetic, developmental, experiential, and serendipitous elements that influence world views, attitudes, and values and ultimately shape illness must be unearthed. Family, education, occupation, and expectations are relevant to a coherent understanding of what the illness means to that person.

The concept of illness offers a useful and pragmatic perspective of diagnosis, not as a label or taxonomic pigeonhole but as the process of receiving, deciphering, and understanding the story of the illness—as narrated from the viewpoint of the individual. The story belongs to the patient and is both a gift and opportunity for the clinician committed to the welfare of that person. In this way, the concept of diagnosis—that is, knowing the causes and contexts for the patient's symptoms and signs—provides the clinician with the requisite information and understanding to recommend a course of management, treatment, and support to alleviate the patient's suffering and ameliorate the loss of function and quality of life stemming from the illness. This broadened diagnostic framework entails understanding the patient's fears, concerns, and desire (or not) for formulations of prognosis and anticipated outcomes. The clinician working with this expansive vantage point of illness is alert to the interactions of the person with family, friends, co-workers, and health care providers and must be attentive, caring, and compassionate. However, it bears reminding that the patient's narrative of illness is readily undermined by the reification of disease and the consequent hijacking of the physician's attention and by the military tropes that often underscore the patient's passivity and render irrelevant the felt experience of illness.

The lack of interest in the patient's narrative is evidenced by the loss and current absence of the voice and words of the patient from the medical case record. This waning of interest did not occur simply because the electronic health record provides few opportunities for the physician's words and reflections on the patient's illness and virtually none for the patient's own words and story. This trend began in the eighteenth century and has accelerated in the twenty-first. The British historian Mary Fissell analyzed physicians' casebooks and revealed that early in the eighteenth century the records included the narrative provided by the patient, often with verbatim descriptions of symptoms and the chronology of the illness. In addition, the case notes included the patient's idiosyncratic explanation of causality and meaning rooted in the person's own particular history and experience. For example, a patient would conclude his symptoms were due to "a chill through incautiously bathing while hot."[6] The physician often accepted and respected these personal, folktale explanations of the sources of illness, basing his diagnosis and treatment on them. By the end of century, however, the narrative is in the words of the doctor and the patient's voice is gone from the casebook. In England in the 1770s, 70 percent of all diagnoses were in English, and 19 percent in Latin. A mere three decades later, "79 percent of all diagnoses were in Latin; only 1 percent were still in English."[7] One reason for this shift of the authorial voice is the changing social roles of doctor and patient. The eighteenth-century physician generally ministered to the well-to-do and was keen to serve the patient well as a continuing source of his livelihood. With the shift to the hospital and the clinic, the agent with greater autonomy was increasingly the physician rather than the patient. With reification of disease and increasing technological complexity, the doctor abducted the narrative and transformed it into a genre not recognizable by patients. The contemporary electronic casebook now reveals only medical jargon and acronyms buttressed by the numbers and images of the medical evidence. Even the physician's words are now sparse.

The loss of the first-person story is emblematic of the transformation of the patient from author and owner of the narrative, whose very particularity served as a means of explicating the mysteries of illness, to a passive, generic, and often solitary bystander and observer of care. The patient's story, especially when validated by the attendant physician, aided in the reduction of uncertainty and served in the construction of meaning, without which the person's experience of illness is fraught with fear and anxiety. All autobiographical descriptions of illness, including those by physicians of their own experiences, describe the loss of control and the disorientation that accompany the inability to participate in the affairs of daily living and the uncertainty that attends the sudden, unexpected onset of illness. In instances where we also expect the patient to be a fighter who must resist being ill, the state of sickness can be complicated by a feeling of having failed to achieve the suitable level of the desire to win. Thus, we compound the injury of disease with the social insult of failure.

An historical analysis by the sociologist N.D. Jewson highlights this loss of not only the patient's voice and narrative but indeed of the person. He traces the phases of medical practice in Europe over the century beginning in 1770 and describes three evolving frameworks: bedside medicine, hospital medicine, and laboratory medicine. In the first phase, medical care was predicated on the "patient's self report of the course of his illness."[8] Over the span of time to 1870, the patient, who began as a person, became a case and then a "cell-complex"; in turn, the physician started as a practitioner, became a clinician, and, finally, a scientist. Jewson thereby describes a transition "away from a person orientated towards an object orientated cosmology."[9] The title of this paper neatly summarizes the point: "The Disappearance of the Sick-Man from Medical Cosmology"—and by the second half of the nineteenth century, the person disappeared "from the medical investigator's field of saliency altogether"[10]—a phenomenon both abetted by and reflected in the prevalent metaphoric discourse.

Blame and Guilt

The sense of guilt imposed on patients is compounded when the disease is situated in a nexus of moral meanings of sin and contagion. The degree of personal responsibility adds to the sense of shame, a sense of guilt laced with a suspicion of transgression: a rather burdensome implicit accusation of self-induced disease with an accompanying whisper of a punishment justly deserved. In the case of cancer, an ancient affliction lacking the explanatory causal mechanisms of infections, the obscure etiologies add to the mystery and darkness of the disease. The sense of evil and mystery and the inexorable advance of the crab of the astrological sign that symbolized cancer was intensified by the framing of moral transgressions and an attendant sense of shame. Little wonder that a finding of cancer was hidden from many patients by their families and caregivers and often went un-named in conversations—as if the word itself had sinister power. Until rather recently, the outcomes of treatments for malignancy were dire, at times underlined by the pessimism of many oncologists. Paradoxically, these same physicians were rather optimistic when raising funds for research and radiated a belief that the disease would eventually be curable. This attitude surely added to the despair sometimes felt by patients and families who could not visualize a personal future of good tidings. Cancer, therefore, replaced the medieval plague as the demonized disease.

Now that intensive research has in fact yielded improvements in survival and slowly decreasing rates of mortality, these metaphoric entailments have diminished, and publicly accessible survivor networks and self-help groups have improved the quality of patients' lives. No longer a secret to be hidden, cancer may lose its dominant position as the evil disease, to be supplanted by a more recent social ill, that of the environmental pollution of the earth, air, and water. To be sure, the sense of immorality has not dissipated but is now shifting to those persons and institutions that despoil and poison nature with toxins and greenhouse gas emissions. The sins of capitalism, modernity, and globalization have spurred a new turn of the ancient cycle.

The concepts of guilt and blame regarding patients, physicians, and diseases have multiple facets that may be parsed linguistically to appreciate their complexities. Once disease is reified, ownership can be assigned to the patient by the physician, as in "your pneumonia" or "the tumor in your belly," or simply assumed by the patient, as in "my high cholesterol" or "my bum ticker" to refer to an arrhythmia. While there is no imputation of immorality or guilt in these semantic formulations, ownership nonetheless implies responsibility. In turn, this engenders a presumption of blame on the part of the innocent patient when things go awry or the treatment fails to achieve its intended result. The language is somewhat different when things go well: physicians are quick to claim victory, as in "my successful treatment" or, more generously at times, "we chose the correct option." By contrast, with lack of success, the physician is more apt to refer to the treatment or opine rather more darkly that the patient was non-compliant and the patient failed chemotherapy. Among the most egregious and colorful of such comments was the report overheard at a gynecology conference that "the patient perforated her uterus on the operating table!"

The articulation of social factors that may contribute to the development of illness can also be (mis-)construed to add to the burden of guilt and blame. For example, poverty, lack of opportunities for education and adequate housing, malnutrition, broken families, and poor drinking water are risk factors for developmental delays of children. These are important issues that demand political solutions and broad-based social change. Yet, all too often, they are mistakenly and carelessly ascribed to poor parental motivation and neglect. Unfortunately, blame is attributed to those who actually require a safety net rather than accusations of apathy and guilt. It is difficult to participate in helpful community action when the outcomes of blame are despair and anger. The point is not that language is responsible for all these societal ills. It is simply that words are used, often unwittingly, to communicate responsibility and guilt and thereby become weapons that exacerbate the problems when they should rather serve as linguistic bearers of support that point to solutions.

The experiences of patients whose illnesses can be traced in part to personal behaviors and modes of living provide another perspective on the continuing moralistic embeddedness of disease in our society. Persons who cope with alcohol or drug abuse, sexually transmitted diseases, or the sequelae of smoking and obesity may face moral opprobrium from friends and health care professionals. As a result, patients need to deal with a sense of blame and perhaps self-retribution that may deplete the requisite resources and motivation for behavioral changes. Persons with other types of illnesses, especially those with mental illnesses, eating disorders, and illnesses with functional disabilities such as fibromyalgia and irritable bowel syndrome that lack traditional pathological evidence of "real" disease may be dismissed as suspected malingerers with such admonitions as "Try harder," "Pull up your socks," and "Get a grip on life." These are, of course, attributions of blame that may emanate from physicians who are frustrated by the demands of caring for patients with complex and poorly understood syndromes. Thus, moral stances underlie the discourse and the clinical mindset. Judgmental frames are also evident in how societies have traditionally dealt geographically with institutions caring for persons with contagious conditions, for example, leprosy and those with severe mental illness. In both instances such facilities were situated well away from other inhabitants and generally outside city limits. While rural settings for those with chronic mental illness or intellectual disabilities may have appeared generously pastoral, the apparent motivation may rather have stemmed from the sad dictum of out of sight, out of mind.

The situation of disease at the nexus of physical purity and moral purity is demonstrated empirically in two interesting papers in experimental psychology exploring the effect of handwashing. Cleanliness and hygiene are important staples of control of infectious diseases in reducing contagion and spread. Similarly, the moral imperative of purity is articulated in the biblical instruction to wash away your sins that gave rise to religious rituals in many different traditions. Zhong and Liljenquist reported in a paper in *Science* that recalling unethical behavior led to "increased mental accessibility of cleansing related concepts"[11] in word completion tasks, and a preference for cleansing products. In addition, a subsequent physical hand cleansing decreased "the upsetting consequence of unethical behavior." A later paper from a different group showed that being asked to recall unethical actions impaired performance on tests of executive control that was "largely eliminated upon wiping hands."[12] Thus, the simple act of handwashing promulgated by all codes of clinical conduct and championed by sanitarian movements has salubrious benefits, both physical and psychological, the latter a result of the deeper metaphysical associations readily evident in language.

An historical, rather than empirical, example of these associations is available in Charles Rosenberg's monograph *The Cholera Years*. He describes that the public health response to the cholera epidemics in the United States insisted on cleanliness as a necessary stance. At the same time, this objective could "call upon those moral energies accumulated by an earlier generation in its struggle for moral salvation.

Personal cleanliness was urged with an almost transcendent zeal; bathing, for example, promised moral as well as physical rewards" and " 'the great washed' " would be " 'the great virtuous.' "[13]

Epidemics Old and New

In January 2020, when a report emerged of an American infected with the newly discovered strain of coronavirus, it took a mere day or so for two Asian-origin high school freshmen in Boston to report being shunned with racist comments from their classmates. Asian university students in Arizona were ostracized by their Caucasian classmates, and the University of California–Berkeley issued a misguided and soon-deleted statement that xenophobia might be a normal reaction to the spread of coronavirus. Within days, the media reported a shadowy announcement that the virus was the creation of rogue Chinese scientists in quest of a bioweapon. While these stories may seem strange, the phenomenon of blame and racism is hardly new or unusual. A professor of history and Asian American studies noted that thinking of Asians as disease carriers is "at least 200 years old" in America and that "this racial story; it's already a part of how you react, and it shows how pervasive it is in our popular culture."[14] In fact, the fear of contagion and pollution and the perceived dangers are evident in very old sources, including the Bible in its description of leprosy and other communicable diseases. This stance of shunning the ill continued to be defended as a societal duty. A nineteenth-century British physician wrote, "The exclusion of lepers from society was considered a high moral duty, simply because the disease was believed to be dreadfully infectious."[15] This fear of the stranger and the other, still evident in the racism elicited during the recent coronavirus epidemics, is dramatically exemplified in the wholesale massacres of Jewish communities in Europe during the Black Death of the mid-fourteenth century. The evil disease that invades from outside miasmas and dirt, both actual and moral, is conflated with strangers and foreigners who are convenient scapegoats and targets in the battle against evil. Blaming the other is evident in the labeling of syphilis as the "French disease" in England, the "Neapolitan disease" in France, the "French evil" in Germany, and the "Christian disease" in Turkey. The term *syphilis* appeared in an epic poem published in Italy in 1530, entitled *Syphilis sive Morbus Gallicus* (Syphilis, or the French Disease).[16,17] Even modern epidemics of influenza carry foreign geographic names rather than neutral labels—to wit, the Spanish influenza pandemic and, more recently, the Hong Kong flu, the Asian flu, West Nile virus, and German measles. By contrast, neither polio nor the swine flu of 2009, both major public health concerns in North America, were ever labeled with American or Canadian place-names.

Many disease legends, including stories of patient-zero for a variety of epidemic outbreaks, express a fear of becoming ill conjoined to an antipathy to outsiders who are considered strange or perverted in some fashion. Both persons and locales that spawned the supposed seed case become stigmatized—while public health workers wish to identify presumed links of contamination and spread of illness, the cultural demand is for an othered or estranged scapegoat. After all, we can only be clean and controlled if an-other is the source of dirt and disorder. Even when the presumed ill person is from within, the language causes social quarantine. Witness the words of a Chinese vice-premier during the events in Wuhan, China, during the COVID outbreak in 2020: "During these wartime conditions, there must be no deserters, or they will be nailed to the pillar of historical shame forever"[18]—a succinct conflation of the metaphor of war, banished deserters, and sacrificial scapegoats expiating our shame. The strength of the nexus between xenophobia and disease is illustrated by the results of an interesting study in social psychology, that those living in an American state with higher rates of infectious diseases exhibited greater degrees of racial prejudices in psychological tests,[19] reminiscent of the historical descriptions that the massacres of innocents during the plague in Europe diminished as the Black Death abated.

Many of the features that characterize the understanding of a developing epidemic and the responses to it, both in speech and in action, are evident in the emergence of AIDS in North America in the 1980s. In a paper that appeared in 1989, Judith Wilson Ross, a medical ethicist, noted that policy discussions around AIDS were infused with and dominated by military language that resulted in the sidelining of those afflicted with the virus: "There is no important role for the sick in a war."[20] The fear, uncertainty, and loss of control led the *New York Times* to reflect the common view that the disease is "an outrage," and such descriptions strengthened the militarized rhetoric evident in professional and lay publications. The linguistic framing led to a trail of consequences that shaped the mindset and thinking about the emerging disease. Congress was asked to declare war on AIDS, others called for a Manhattan Project, and potential casualties were compared to military losses in the Korean and Vietnam Wars. Ross points out that war demands an enemy—in the first instance, the responsible virus, and secondarily, those who harbor the virus or are described as carriers. She notes that the word *harbor* is used to describe those who protect an enemy and are thus akin to spies and traitors. An obvious question for states of war is, "Who caused the conflict?" This generated an intensive search for patient-zero, and one AIDS researcher referred to this as a question of "original sin."[21] The widely described suspects were geographic or social foreigners, namely, Cubans, Haitians, Africans, or gay men, in other words, "groups already stigmatized in the US." Ross also underscored the moral overtones of the contemporary debate by presciently noting that "American wars are always holy wars and righteous wars, and a war on AIDS will inevitably be translated into attitudes of punishment and justice."[22] It is sobering to recall the proposals in the 1980s for the tattooing of those found to be infected with the virus as part of public health policy. While we may now believe that we have transcended such draconian measures, the anxious daily press reports of the coronavirus outbreak belie such optimism.

Sanitarian Movements

The mandate of clinical medicine is the care of the individual patient and family unit, while epidemics and the advent of broadened notions of risk factors and complex causalities spurred the development of the discipline of public health with its attention to the welfare of entire communities and populations. This became a professional pursuit with medical officers of health and schools of public health, in both North America and Europe. In addition, there were initiatives concerned with the modern analogs of medieval miasmas, swamp fevers, and invisible influences that developed before the discoveries of Pasteur, Koch, and the pioneers of bacteriology. These broad social movements involved many actors in addition to physicians and included broad representation from members of the public, educational institutions, politicians, philanthropists, and religious organizations. Interesting examples include Florence Nightingale's work in the Crimean War and her role in the sanitarian movement in England of the middle of the nineteenth century, spurred in part by the horrific loss of life due to defective hygiene and sanitation services in the theater of war. In turn, this inspired the creation during the American Civil War of the United States Sanitary Commission, dedicated to the care of soldiers of the Union army. These entities, organized originally to respond to the conditions on the battlefields and in military and, later, civilian hospitals, soon became active social movements in Britain and the United States with a direct interest in the conditions of cleanliness and hygiene in the community and the home. These sanitary movements illustrated the influences of militarized language and the cultural linkage between disease and morality already evident in traditional medicine. They serve as examples of how the leitmotifs of battle and sin shaped public health as they had previously inflected the behaviors of patients and physicians.

The important work by Bruno Latour on the influence of Pasteur on medicine and the hygienist movement in France is entitled *Les Microbes: Guerre et Paix* (the English translation is *The Pasteurization of France*). His introduction states as follows: "The Pasteur blitzkrieg, in striking contrast to the physicians' and surgeons' blind struggle against an invisible enemy, reveals a convincing scientific manner, free of compromise, tinkering, and controversy."[23] It entails wars and struggles against powerful enemies, presumably the soon-to-be discovered germs. The use of moral and religious imagery in public health is most readily appreciated in the sanitary institutions in the United States, as described by Nancy Tomes and foreshadowed in the title of her book, *The Gospel of Germs*. The various associations and institutions that comprised the sanitarian movements in the United States made liberal use of biblical sources for moral suasion and organized troops to self-describe their valiant efforts to ensure the purity of hearth, home, the workplace, and the public square. As noted, "The sanitarian crusade was couched in religious as well as scientific terms" and preached "a sanitary gospel of redemptive cleanliness."[24]

Two examples will illustrate the rhetorical stances evident in the historical sources presented by Tomes. An emphasis on personal cleanliness and on the home, together with a desire to enlist community, nonprofessional volunteers, led to the centrality of attention to women, especially housewives and mothers. A book on personal hygiene reminded its female readers that "cleanliness is the outward sign of inner purity"[25] and women were assured that housework is "a sort of religion, a step in the conquering of evil, for dirt is sin."[26] The housewife's "Mosaic code"[27] included "obedience to sanitary laws," with special attention to the "recesses" of the refrigerator that were sure to "hide a multitude of sins." Not surprisingly, such movements "inevitably increased the stigmatization of the sick and poor" and abetted "nativists and racists"[28] who were committed to barring entry to immigrants. Indeed, the United States sharply reduced immigration in 1924, as these sanitarian movements were gaining supporters and energy. At the same time, the abodes of the wealthy were not spared the wrath of the sanitarian evangelists. Tomes cites the pithy descriptor "whited sepulchers"[29] that appeared in 1883 in an article entitled "The Unsanitary Homes of the Rich," referring to the posh Manhattan homes of the well-to-do. This relies on a New Testament reference to "Pharisees who, like a whitewashed tomb that disguised the decaying bodies inside, appeared righteous, but actually were riddled with sin." Thus, the very wealthy, much like the highly impoverished, needed "hygienic redemption."[30]

The challenges were equally great for mothers. A pamphlet promulgated by the New York Bureau of Child Hygiene, entitled *The Ten Commandments for Keeping Baby Well*, described the "three deadly D's, Disease, Dirt and Death"[31] and exhorted mothers to counter these with "the three C's, Cleanliness, Comfort and Contentment." These emphases on child-rearing, cleanliness, and the home added to the burden on women for whom "this new knowledge brought both a new sense of power and a heavy load of guilt." Where sin may be found, guilt cannot be far removed. To strengthen the will and endurance of these female fighters, they were reminded of their special duties by a Cornell home economist (a woman): "You have your battles to fight every day and I believe that when a woman does this well, she is as much of a heroine as the soldier is a hero on the battlefield."[32] One can easily imagine that if family members succumbed to tuberculosis, these burdened women were stricken with guilt. It is important to recall that these moral exhortations and expressions of fervor are gleaned from materials that appeared in late nineteenth-century America, not from medieval or Puritan sources, though the language is clearly the same.

A second heuristic example documented by Tomes is the social response to tuberculosis, the endemic and devastating illness that spread by community contact. The anti-tuberculosis social campaign had the "fervor of a new religion" that claimed that "spitting was indecent" and "a mortal sin."[33] The moral characterization continued with the comments that the tubercle bacillus had "Satanic power." Public awareness campaigns included tracts and pamphlets that recalled evangelical movements with lists of commandments and catechisms, and the Edison Film Company released an educational feature film entitled *The Temple of Moloch*, warning the public of the dangers of community dissemination of tuberculosis. These community efforts culminated in the founding of The National Tuberculosis Association (NTA), which soon gained the support of three American presidents and launched over a thousand chapters and many thousands of volunteers across the country. At its second annual meeting, in 1906, the Association adopted as its official emblem the double-barred cross, whose design was modeled on the Lorraine Cross that had been chosen by Godfrey, Duke of Lorraine, a leader of the first Crusade as his standard when he became ruler of Jerusalem in 1099. This cross became well known in Europe during the Crusades, and this religious-military standard was proudly displayed on the helmets and capes of the children enrolled as crusader members of the Modern Health Crusade promulgated by the NTA. The young volunteers were assigned ranks from squire to knight at the table of "Health Chivalry" depending on their talent at raising funds. The Modern Health Crusade, reflecting its inspiration by the medieval crusades, spurred one young participant to note that "the germs are the Turks."[34] A rather pithy allusion to a religiously inspired holy war directed against a modern bacterial infidel.

Prevention

The reification of disease undermined the understanding of disease as a biological process whose development and course depended on a host of contextual host and environmental factors.[35] Diagnosis thereby became a detective search for the locus of disease, the causal agent, and its mode of access to the body. In the same vein, prevention is framed as the means of blocking access to invaders and is rooted in creating barriers to immigration of agents of disease by a variety of public health interventions. At times, as we have seen during epidemics, the fear of an infectious organism is conferred on human immigrants or others who are considered the carriers. Thus, border patrols can be both literal and metaphoric, and what should be a logical, thoughtful, and data-driven analysis of a diversity of risk factors becomes a chaotic, panic-driven response under conditions of stress and fear. This may be accompanied by anxious and hurried efforts to create a vaccine whose urgency is forgotten once the danger has abated. With diminished fear and fading memories, the necessary funds vanish, and all work is abandoned until the next crisis erupts. Prevention becomes a response to an evident or imminent threat when the World Health Organization (WHO) raises the level of alert, much like the military in reaction to an impending missile strike. In neither threat, that of pandemic or global war, is the lessening of urgency accompanied by consideration of ecological responses in the first case or political negotiations in the second. Rather than pursue what appears to be the boring work of planning and prevention, the decisions often appear to be to wait for the next crisis, with its rush of adrenalin and its demand for action. After all, when the framing in both cases is to fight the invader, a metaphoric battle in the one and an actual war in the latter, other responses do not appear cogent. More sober forms of illness prevention with consistent attention to the social determinants of health—namely, sanitation, nutrition, relief of poverty on a population basis—and accompanied by diet, exercise, and stress reduction on a personal level are not accommodated comfortably by a military model. Moreover, the latter demands action against an enemy, not reflections on how to diminish risks to the body-human or the body-politic. Prevention cannot readily be understood as a war and does not generate broad attention within the predominant cultural model. In this sense, public health becomes a poor relation by a process similar to that which renders chronic illness less captivating than acute conditions, certainly in the minds of many physicians and, perhaps, even for some patients. After all, when all is said and done, military leaders are most at home on fields of battle, politicians are responsive to short timelines, and Western medicine is attuned to acute illnesses and heroic interventions. Effective preventive measures cannot be readily construed as war—they do not generate rapid returns and rapt attention and are thus of diminished interest. Our metaphors guide our predilections and deciphering them helps us understand our choices. The resultant clarity may offer different pathways to health, sanitation, and sanity.

Military metaphors undermine effective preventive measures for communities and populations by pointing to adversarial measures rather than programs of cleanliness and avoidance. Concurrently, such language has deleterious consequences for individual behaviors. Hauser and Schwarz designed psychological experiments to elucidate the effects of linguistic priming on personal decisions when faced with behavioral choices and options. They tested the effect of metaphorically framing cancer as an enemy on participant responses. They measured a reduction in the conceptual accessibility of self-limiting preventive measures and a decrease in participants' intentions to adopt putatively beneficial behaviors. The study was based on the hypothesis that many preventive measures require a stance of avoidance rather than action, for example, smoking, alcohol, and sun exposure. However, a militarized response emphasizes "masculinity and taking aggressive actions toward an enemy"[36]—all antithetical to behaviors "which entail limitation and restraint." A second study[37] by the same investigators demonstrated that presenting cancer contextualized within war metaphors increased the perceived difficulties of treatments and led to more fatalistic beliefs regarding malignancies. Contrary to expectations, such military metaphors did not make subjects more likely to seek advice regarding a suspicious finding, for example, a breast or testicular lump. Thus, and perhaps paradoxically, a cancer diagnosis may call for a war and induce a loss of hope exacerbated by a fatalism, yet fail to spur individuals to seek timely advice, thereby delaying potentially helpful treatments. Preventive measures, whether at a broad social policy level or within the personal medical setting, are undermined by the battle and war metaphors, as such avoidance behaviors are at odds with the entrenched exhortations to fight at all costs.

An interesting dimension of the interplay of the military framework and differing models of prevention is provided by an analysis by Alfred Tauber on the evolving understandings of the immune system in human biology and identity.[38] A traditional conception viewed the human as an autonomous individual protected by immune defenses against a world of foreign others and invaders seeking to attack and destroy the self. The immune system distinguishes self from non-self and launches multi-pronged attacks on the latter. This is consonant with the description of military metaphors underwriting the macho, individualistic, and aggressive image of a fighter at risk from the surrounding world of alien non-selfs. By contrast, a more recent framing understands the human in a relational, ecological dialogue with the greater biological and social worlds, both internal and outer. This envisions an immune system with an evolving and fluid notion of what is potentially harmful in a specific context and point in time. For example, the microbiome that is part of the internal and surface milieu of all persons is essential to the function of the gut, the brain, and normal development. Thus, while non-self, the microbiome is hardly an enemy—rather a symbiont than an invader. Military language and cognition are barriers to a new relational, ecological conception of what is means to be human and a self that is integrated within a broad biopsychosocial world of organisms.

Therapy

The militarized notion of disease and medicine reshapes the aims and modes of treatment as it inflects our understanding of diagnostics, epidemics, and prevention. If the state of health and well-being is tantamount to an absence of war and a condition of peace, then the aim of therapy is complete conquest and elimination of disease. Furthermore, as disease and sin are related, medical ritual should lead to physical restoration and to the state antecedent to illness, just as religious ritual provides absolution and return to a state of moral purity. However, while medical interventions often bring relief, remission, and diminished angst and suffering, they are only rarely capable of eradicating all signs of disease from the body and mind. Even successfully managed acute conditions such as infections and fractures leave residua of calluses and scars and, perhaps more optimistically, a more robust immune response the second time around. The body and its immune and nervous systems and the mind all have memories, some helpful and others traumatic. Thus, while illness may indeed abate and resolve, the sequelae of disease remain. The situation is even more complex in the case of chronic illnesses, whose prevalence is increasing rapidly. While such conditions are highly amenable to management by medical and allied health professionals and can settle into long remissions, the underlying causality and disease processes may not disappear. One can control and mitigate hypertension and reduce blood pressure to normal levels with ongoing treatments, but the disease cannot be extirpated and removed. Rheumatoid arthritis, coronary insufficiency, and inflammatory bowel disease are currently responsive to new pharmacological interventions and supportive care to the point where patients carry on normal lives with little functional impairment. However, these results are due to careful, painstaking adjustments and incremental improvements in a collaboration between patient and physician and not the outcome of a victory of militarized physicians over mortal enemies. The current and indeed successful practice of medicine is neither well described nor well served by the traditional models and entrenched language.

In fact, the old construct may even undermine important aspects of therapeutic practice. By imagining health as an Edenic state, and the aim of medicine as complete restoration, we promote a misleading and inappropriate objective. This anticipated and hoped-for outcome underwrites a mindset of conquest, the reluctance to seek truces, never-ending treatments and attempts at cure, and a warlike stance such that a shift from curative to palliative care is somehow a surrender to the enemy. Little wonder that a large proportion of health care expenditures are dedicated to acute care in the remaining months of life and that most novel cancer drugs in clinical trials are designed to deal with metastatic disease and offer small increments of survival. Two other consequences are noteworthy: the few situations where physicians might lay claim to total victory are acute diseases—hence, chronic illnesses are less interesting and receive less funding and research support. Second, necessary alliances between patient and physician are less common in acute interventions in which patients tend to be passive recipients of care. One may even surmise that physicians engaged in mortal combat do not view patients as natural allies, underscoring the concept of the patient as the field of battle.

A Reversal of Roles

The moral embeddedness of disease points to a number of parallels between physicians and priests. While the noun *minister* is ordinarily used to refer to a member of the clergy, the OED cites a sixteenth-century usage as "a person who administers medicine; a physician."[39] The verb *to minister* is defined both as "to serve or officiate at a religious service" and "to apply or administer (medicine, poison)"[40] and in both instances "to be of help, comfort, or service to" a parishioner or a patient. In the earliest examples of the religion–medicine interface, the dominant persona with healing powers was the ecclesiastical figure following the biblical and Augustinian framing of Christ the Physician. The priest performed the rituals for forgiveness and absolution, and the resultant spiritual healing was followed by bodily cures. The mystery of the process added to its power and carried with it the magic of ancient shamanic interventions. By contrast, physicians of the day were hardly exalted figures and were providers of poultices, potions, and blood-letting.

Until the mid-eighteenth century, doctors were medical servants to the wealthy rather than greatly respected members of society. The apparatus of salvation was under the aegis of the priesthood in its various guises, depending on time and place. Since then, there has been a role reversal and shift of the hierarchy. As organized religion has waned in importance in contemporary societies, the practice of medicine assumed responsibility for the magic and ritual, and physicians began a long rise in societal status and importance starting in the late eighteenth century. Today, physicians are seen as more powerful than priests in their impact on the lives and well-being of persons. Scientific developments and technological improvements have made possible treatments that might have been understood as miracles a millennium earlier. Organ transplantation, in vitro fertilization, robotic surgery, and engineered replacements for sensory losses, to name only a few, are the salvations of the new millennium. Gene manipulation by CRISPR molecular surgery is laced with mystery and unknowable dangers but is already described with promises of mythic proportions. Physicians and their technological allies have now taken on Christ-like powers of resurrection with prospects of biblical-scale longevities. On a less dramatic but no less impressive canvas, the body has gained a new sanctity, with bariatric surgery and cosmetic implants, and Botox injections as the new holy water—hardly the spiritual temple of the past, but a form of worship all the same. Even the healing power of the confessional has been supplanted by television therapists, public witnessing, and tell-all reality shows. While the forms have changed, what remains recognizable is the power of ritual, magic, and morality.

New Recruits

As we look ahead, two developments appear imminent: personalized/genomic medicine and robots/artificial intelligence (AI). We live in a time heralded as the golden age of personalized medicine in which individual-specific genetic and other risk factors are analyzed to pinpoint diagnoses and customize therapies. Such approaches are showing promise in permitting more refined and appropriate interventions. At the same time, we witness an explosion of interest in genetic identity and ancestry as a source of pride with a burgeoning interest in genetic factors in causality for various ills, both actual and predicted. Together, there is a broad popular attention to genetics not seen since the 1920s and '30s. This may present a two-fold risk. One is a shift of emphasis away from environmental, social, and cultural factors in disease and illness toward a more reductionist gene-centered notion of causality. The second is perhaps more germane to our subject matter of agency and guilt. That is, if persons celebrate their genetic endowments and ancestries, they may concurrently begin to feel guilt and familial blame for inherited mutations and other genetic contributions to risk. It is important for physicians to help patients avert both misconceptions—namely, that there is a gene for beauty, intelligence, and other socially desired traits, and second, that aberrant genes that increase risk are somehow the fault of the carrier rather than a serendipitous mutation or other untoward event in the economy and regulation of the genome. Both misconceptions lead to false understandings and promote once again old notions of destiny and morality.

We will soon witness the addition of new recruits to the military medical armory, namely, robotic and AI systems in fighting disease. These are of three general types. The first is AI software designed to scan data sets of one or more patients to spot significant changes or trends that may escape a cursory review by a busy practitioner. More sophisticated versions incorporating neural networks can be employed to assist physicians in suggesting diagnostic possibilities. Imaging systems analyze, for example, routine X-rays, screening mammograms, and skin conditions to spot important anomalies and lesions and can do so at a speed not possible for human observers. Finally, surgical robots directed by surgeons sitting at consoles remote from the patient and operative field may improve delicate and finely controlled surgical procedures. While the surgeon controls and directs the movements of the robotic arms and instruments, the distance from the patient is now unlimited, so that the actual human operator may be situated remotely, from five feet to thousands of miles away. Some technological experts foresee the development of surgeon-less robots, akin to driverless cars. This is somewhat analogous to military drones piloted from afar that later gain decision-making capacity to independently choose suitable targets.

Such technical marvels may indeed improve the quality of care and perhaps even improve outcomes, though such benefits await rigorous clinical trials. Nonetheless, our concern is the arrival of a new entity intercalated between physician and patient, thus decreasing the direct human interaction necessary for optimal care, while increasing the passivity of the recipient patient, newly attended by robotic caregivers. A Luddite response opposing the introduction of new computer-based technologies is clearly inappropriate. However, it will be relevant and necessary to carefully examine the effects of such devices on patients to ensure that their sense of connection and trust in their attending clinicians is not impaired by these robotic strangers at the bedside.

7

Resilience of Military Metaphors

I can't let cancer kill me until both my knowledge of it and my work on the new book is done. I have to keep going even if all the odds are against me. Somehow, someway, I will win. I will ... I'm going to beat this thing.... I won't be beaten.

—Cornelius Ryan, *A Private Battle*

The longevity and ubiquity of the language of battle and war in public and clinical discourse prompt us to consider the benefits that these metaphors provide that might explain their widespread use. After all, staying power over millennia suggests their usefulness for some speakers and thinkers, especially in medical contexts. Examples noted in earlier chapters have described the untoward effects of these metaphors on the thoughts and behaviors of patients and physicians and on their interactions. Yet, perhaps there are settings where and persons for whom such tropes are helpful. Talk of the military evokes power, victory, and a stance of control and self-reliance. The fighter is characterized by a will to win, at times at all costs, and this persona may be attractive to patients for whom figures of war and victory are particularly relevant and resonant. Some who served in the military and in combat have memories of camaraderie and freedom from quotidian responsibilities and find the language of war and service reassuring. Others, who may not have shared such experiences, may nonetheless be most comfortable with the sense of control and personal responsibility. Military metaphors infuse and color the daily events for some patients as they deal with grave illness.

A Private Battle

Cornelius Ryan was a war correspondent who reported on the US Army in Europe during World War II. He later become a well-known and highly regarded chronicler of the war in Europe through a series of books, including *The Longest Day*, describing the Allied landings on D-Day in 1944, and *A Bridge Too Far*, telling the story of the disastrous Allied foray to enter Germany in late 1944. While he was about to launch the writing of the latter volume in 1970, Ryan was diagnosed with prostate cancer, and his experiences of the illness and patienthood are eloquently told in the book,

A Private Battle, published after his death. The pathography—an illness biography or autobiography by patients and/or their families—comprises Ryan's contemporaneous notes and audio diary he produced over a four-year period between diagnosis and death, together with the diary of his wife, Kathryn Morgan, and various medical records and materials she later compiled and annotated.

Ryan frames his four-year experience of illness as a war and the chapter headings as a series of military maneuvers, including "The Plan," "The Attack," and "The Battle."[1] In her work on pathographies, Ann Hunsaker Hawkins describes Ryan's narrative as an exemplar of the warrior patient, the link between Ryan as war correspondent and as patient is an "aggressive determination, an attitude and an ideal which is modeled upon the heroic World War II soldiers of Arnhem and Nijmegen"[2] [two epic battles detailed in *A Bridge Too Far*]. Not surprisingly, Ryan relies on the reified construct of disease that "cancer will be my closest possession"[3] and contrasts his experiences in the war with his challenges as patient: "This battle is immediate. I'm squarely in the middle of it and my knowledge of the enemy's strength and probable movements is, as of this moment, pathetically slim."[4] In keeping with his career as a journalist and chronicler, he initiates a process of information gathering (reconnaissance) and seeks referrals to well-known urologists in order to define his plan of attack, not defense, against a disease that would become "a tangible murderer, stalking his every move."[5] His meetings with physicians are "combat councils"[6] and, as Hawkins notes, for Ryan, the doctors "are reminiscent of the various generals of World War II about whom he writes in his histories."[7] She then extends the metaphor as follows: "His cancer is of course the enemy, the therapies function as weaponry, and the many helpful friends are like the courageous civilians of the Resistance. Ryan himself figures in this private allegory not only as the battlefield upon which rage those forces of the disease and the therapy, but also as a commander-in-chief in consultation with other generals (his physicians) planning the battle."[8] Ryan is not simply a fighter who plans to win but also the supreme commander of the war. Not a lone participant and certainly not a passive observer, he is fully engaged and is awake the night before his surgery for, after all, "on the eve of battle ... no one really sleeps."[9]

What Hawkins calls a "private allegory" carries through the surgery and postoperative period. As Ryan writes, "I remember that when I came to after the operation I thought I had been badly wounded in the war. There appeared to be bottles and tubes all around me, and to my mind these are synonymous with the equipment used by medics in the field."[10] Ryan describes his postop pain "as though a half-track has rolled back and forth across my stomach non-stop for several days," and his assessment of the operation is a commander's report: "The attack was successful, although I am expecting a counter-attack any moment from all sides."[11] The theme of battle thoroughly infuses and gives meaning to Ryan's mode of coping with his illness. As his wife, who described herself as joining Ryan in "the foxhole,"[12] notes, "He had never intended to give up without a fight. His unyielding nature was his best medicine and his strongest ally."[13] Ryan sees himself as the major protagonist of the battle with cancer and thereby gains agency and a sense of control. Passivity is anathema to him, and when a noted urologist suggests an approach of watchful waiting, his patient is taken aback and replies, "Doctor, one can't imagine doing absolutely nothing."[14] Ryan demands active interventions and declines a prolonged course of radiotherapy, as it entails nine weeks of passivity and patience.

The role of patient is, for Ryan, accompanied by a loss of dignity and pride that is, in part, countered by the stance of control and agency. On admission to hospital he is asked to undress and describes himself as "defenseless.... You aren't a person any longer. You're a patient—without dignity or sense of self. There's no way to keep your guard up."[15] For Ryan as fighter, the "kingdom of the ill" is both a strange and threatening land. When visiting a radiotherapy waiting room, he observes the guide markers tattooed on patients that indicate "the areas in which cancer could and does strike, leaving human beings without dignity, exposing their vulnerability for everyone to see."[16] The perceived assault by the tumor and the loss of personhood is soon exacerbated by the added loss of masculinity resulting from hormonal therapy, and later by muscle weakness, an inability to walk, incontinence, and the loss of individuality. When asked to complete hospital forms, Ryan observes, "You're nothing but one piece of rice in a vast rice field to be tabulated."[17] He offers a poignant description of the demands faced by a person who opts to fight and strives to prevail: "While I believe that 90 percent of the battle resides in one's positive state of mind and a strong determination to win, willpower and mood are constantly undermined by cancer. It erodes not only the body but dignity and self-respect. The most difficult art to perfect is the art of being ill gracefully."[18] Ryan abhors the "self-pity" that may attend "the plague of chronic illness" and prefers the challenge of physical pain. The metaphor of a warrior battling with cancer provides for Ryan a perspective laden with meaning that shapes his attitude and behavior and provides imagery that brings its own values and benefits. As Hawkins observes, "the battle myth is consciously used as an actual therapeutic device"[19] and "myth has become medicine." For Ryan, with his lived experiences and framework of values, the battle myth makes possible "some transcendence over his illness."[20] It inspired the note that Ryan left for his surgeon the night before surgery, based on a description of the D-Day landing: "They flashed the signal everyone would remember this night—3 dots and a dash. The V for Victory."[21]

However valiant the fight and brave the fighter, it becomes increasingly clear to Ryan that victory is not to be. Ryan does not abandon the metaphor of war but shifts to a different image of combat: no longer a tactical commander, he is an ordinary soldier whose virtues are courage, determination, and a desire to maintain dignity and resolve to the last. He believes that "courage is at its peak when one has run out of hope,"[22] and the need to stay the course is reflected in a fear of introspection: "I must take care not to turn inward.... It would, I think, be an almost certain sign that subconsciously I was giving up."[23] Despite this aversion, he offers two remarkable observations: "Strange to say, there is a virtue in having cancer. It makes one more sensitive to others,"[24] and "There can be no understanding of war or disease without knowledge of what the individuals involved endured."[25] Finally, Ryan intertwines his oeuvre as a war correspondent and author and his life as a patient in an epitaphic phrase: "It is his [the writer's] privilege to help man endure by lifting his heart, by reminding him of the courage and honor and hope and pride and compassion and pity and sacrifice which have been the glory of his past."[26]

For Cornelius Ryan, the battle metaphor serves as an adaptable framework for action and provides a sense of agency and control that is a counterpoint to the usual passivity of patienthood. It encompasses both the role of the winning commander and the undaunted courageous soldier when faced with defeat. The heroic stance entails dignity, pride, and masculinity resonant with Ryan's identity and career. The fighter's attitude is also empowering, as Hawkins points out, because it is "medically syntonic; that is, consistent with the metaphors and myths inherent in western medicine."[27] Most of the physicians and surgeons Ryan meets are themselves enculturated in a militaristic understanding of their craft, with the exception of the lone urologist who counsels watchful waiting and evokes a sense of dismay in his patient. As Hawkins underlines, "Myths about illness not only reflect experience but they also determine its actual shape."[28]

We now live and work in a linguistic landscape in which more medicine is preferred to less, aggressive therapies are celebrated, where fighters, whether physicians or patients, or military leaders believe victory is inevitable and every war is righteous. Yet, even for Ryan, the belief exacts a price—the shame of a cancer diagnosis prevents him from sharing the news with good friends and necessitates the bravado and camouflage for his vulnerability. He suffers pain for many months but declines medication, explaining that "I am neither at peace nor without pain when I am well."[29] Later on, with his book completed, Ryan still declines to rest, opining, "Somehow I feel that inactivity and leisure time would give cancer an edge."[30] Health and illness both mean constant determination and striving to be better. Those are precisely the values that infuse Ryan's sense of the world and his self within it and delineate the powerful myth that provides meaning and the trajectory of his life.

Hawkins presents a second pathography, *Heartsounds*, authored by Martha Lear, whose husband, a surgeon, required major surgery for severe heart disease. He, too, was a person attuned to the battle metaphor and an aggressive approach to dealing with illness. She describes a postoperative nightmare that spurred her husband to awake suddenly with the exclamation, "Where is my adversary?"[31] Lear notes her husband's "neat surgical mind demanding an adversary, an enemy, a pathology, recognizable forces of death and disease against which he might pit his own skills."[32] He, too, needs a reified disease as an opponent and target for battle, but his heart could not be readily construed as an enemy. The pathography goes on to document the patient's "confusion and deepening despair" and the author's "rage and helplessness"[33] at her husband's plight.

Hawkins draws a contrast between Ryan and Lear as patients. The military language was consonant with both the war correspondent and the surgeon. But while this trope serves as an "enabling myth"[34] for the journalist, it fails to provide comfort for the surgeon. Lear's inability to abandon this frustrating and tormenting frame led to anger and suffering. Hawkins differentiates an enabling military myth from one that fails. To provide support and value for the patient, the metaphor requires an identifiable adversary as the target for aggression and anger. The person who is the patient and commander must have like-minded allies—physicians who share the metaphoric mindset of battle. And, suitable weapons should be at hand. Only then can there be a possibility of victory and the battle myth can underwrite the requisite sense of control and strength. In the case of the surgeon Lear, his failing heart was not an enemy, his doctors did not see themselves as allies in a war, and there were few weapons to combat either the cardiac disease or the array of major postoperative complications. While both patients succumbed to their illnesses, Ryan died a courageous fighter hero, and Lear died in anger. This sharp difference of experience highlights the Janus-like nature of the war metaphor. As Hawkins notes, "The war metaphor always seems to imply some degree of ambivalence, perhaps because it embodies both the glory of heroism and the horror of suffering and death"[35]—much like war itself.

The realization that the battle metaphor may be helpful for some patients and detrimental to others presents an added mandate for physicians providing care for patients with severe and chronic illnesses. The variability may stem from personality differences and character traits, may reflect the life experiences that shape mindsets and viewpoints, and the nature of the illness itself can motivate different needs. Both Ryan and Lear saw themselves as fighters, yet the specific contexts were strikingly dissimilar. Tumors are readily reified enemies, Ryan's physicians shared his mindset, and surgery was a suitable weapon of attack for the planned extirpation of the foe. Lear's massive myocardial infarction left a weakened heart that was hardly a satisfactory target of war, and the many difficulties and complications of his postoperative care did not recruit his physicians as allies. Finally, there were not many pharmacological, let alone surgical, weapons available to grapple with a failing heart.

The situation becomes more complex when the framework that may help the patient during the course of illness changes with time, context, and stage of illness. Hawkins recounts a story of a couple with AIDS whose joint response to illness was a desire to fight—to seek a "magic bullet" with a military stance to fend off "despair." The unfortunate corollary to maintaining a battle attitude beyond the point at which it may have been helpful becomes evident when that stance becomes "disabling." The plan to win at all costs is accompanied by an intense denial of the possibility of loss. This denial blinded the two individuals to the impending end, and the survivor mourned the lost opportunity to share their feelings and goodbyes. As Hawkins summarizes, "Given the degree of denial, which seems quite probably a function of the strength of the military myth, this proved impossible."[36] A framework that serves to shore up hope and optimism at one stage of illness may cause suffering at a later phase. The battle perspective may be so engrained societally and individually as to be nigh on impossible to abandon or reframe.

The Athletic Fighter

The heroic athlete, a strong figure in both ancient Greece and today's Western societies, is characterized by a desire to win, play "hard," and fight to the end. Athletes, both men and women, are now celebrated almost universally and are handsomely rewarded with fame and fortune and recognized as heroes. The concept of winning the game is often used during illness by men and women for whom sports are important to their daily interests and concerns, whether as actual participants or fanatic observers and followers of the sports pages of newspapers and websites. The discourse of the world of sports offers up fighting metaphors of striving, competing, and winning. Attitude and mindset are lauded by sports psychologists, both professional and amateur, and instill a sense of control and self-reliance and the pride of can-do. Getting better is crossing the goal line, scoring a touchdown, or a race to the finish. The doctor's proposal for therapy is the "game plan," and a consultation is the "huddle." Prognoses are couched in terms of odds and probabilities as in a Las Vegas sports casino and a "long-shot" is aspirational rather than predictive. Patients with later stages of illness seek an unexpected "hole-in-one," a "grand slam home-run," a "Hail Mary pass," and endeavor "to cross the finish line by a nose."

For patients keen on sports, these tropes provide a familiar discourse to replace the strange and technical language of disease and the clinic. Men often feel restrained and intimidated by sharing details of their concerns and fears for themselves, their families, and their futures, and sports-talk offers an alternative mode of communication. Viewing the threat of disease as a challenging contest provides some distance from what can be a harsh reality and serves as a buffer against despair. The notion of being a player or the quarterback is akin to the military commander and affords a sense of being in charge and averts the common passivity of patienthood. Nonetheless, beyond the evident similarities between the soldier and the athlete, there are helpful and perhaps comforting distinctions. As Hawkins points out, the challenge in the war metaphor is the enemy—disease—whereas the challenge for the athlete is the self: to be the best that one can be. The imperative is striving to win by gaining control over one's own limitations. Rather than the unequal fight against a ruthless enemy faced by a soldier, the athlete relies on a personal mindset and skills to win the game. And, if winning proves impossible, at the least one can choose to lose with dignity, having exerted the supreme effort. The sports metaphor retains the possibility and aspirational goal of victory and may also avert guilt, blame, and despair. Just as the military fight may end with a heroic soldier, the athletic game can result in a gracious loser. Both soldiers and athletes are respected for fighting to the last, whether on the fields of war or the fields of play.

Sports metaphors can be helpful to athletes, sports fans, and perhaps children and teenagers dealing with serious illness, and the tropes work well when patients are improving. However, the implicit denial of the serious nature of illness by the belief that losing a game may simply entail planning for the following match or the next season can become a barrier to coping with a diminishing prognosis. The challenge, as in the instance of battle metaphors, is to appreciate when they evolve from helpful to harmful. Once again, the shift adds to the duties of physicians who must understand the rapidly changing contexts for their patients and provide guidance and support for those with severe illness who may be understandably confused and fearful when their figurative underpinnings are stripped bare. Even for those for whom one might presume a metaphor of striving and fighting would be helpful—for example, an outstanding athlete—thoughtful clinical attention is crucial. Reisfield and Wilson cite the instance of Lance Armstrong, a renowned cycling champion and celebrated sports hero, who was advised by an oncologist to accept a very aggressive chemotherapy regimen for a newly discovered malignancy. The physician, either because of his own understanding of the oncologist's role as a military commander, or in response to the athletic reputation of his patient, chose a rather unfortunate rhetorical presentation as follows: "I'm going to kill you. Every day, I'm going to kill you, and then I'm going to bring you back to life. We're going to hit you with chemo, and then hit you again, and hit you again. You're not going to be able to walk. We're practically going to have to teach you to walk again after we're done."[37] The rather stunned patient described his response to this manifestly violent recommendation as "shell shock," and promptly left that treatment center to seek care elsewhere. This error and insensitivity by a clinician presuming that a particular persona, say soldier or athlete, would necessarily respond well to the language of war is sobering and cautionary.

The Fighting Physician

Patients may take on or be co-opted into the role of protagonists in the battle against disease. In other instances, physicians are the commanders and military leaders in the metaphoric wars. A take-charge physician who assumes control and is ready to make decisions may be a helpful and comforting figure to a patient and family who place their trust in a surrogate in the battle. The complexity of various diagnostic and therapeutic modalities afforded by biomedical science hastened the progression of the trusted caregiver from paternalistic family physician to technologically savvy specialist. The advent of robotic surgery, stereotactic radiation, and customized biological therapies has necessitated detailed technical knowledge and the control of daunting machinery. Increasingly, patients feel secure in assigning responsibility to physicians and are thereby spared the need to expend energy on deciphering complex guidelines and a Sargasso Sea of recommendations and choices. Given the common notion that diseases, whether malignant, infectious, epidemic, inflammatory, or psychiatric, are foreign entities intruding on the body and mind, it is understandable that a patient and family are reassured by a militant doctor. Indeed, there may be consolation in ceding authority to the physician as fighter who can be a source of security compared to one who defers to the authority of patients but abdicates the duty to inform and guide complex choices. A doctor who declares to a patient that "the decisions are yours to make" may err in respecting a person's autonomy at the cost of creating confusion and fear.

William May, in his book entitled *The Physician's Covenant*, provides a nuanced and instructive typology of military models by referring to the heroic generals of WWII.[38] For example, General George Patton was a daring and bold commander but demanded absolute control with a "Caesarean view of military command." Field Marshal Bernard Montgomery was brilliant in strategy but hampered by "a vanity that clouded his judgment in collaborative enterprises." The more modest General Omar Bradley appeared to be a "more attractive alternative mixing competence and teamwork and a sense for the limits of one's authority." Not surprisingly, fighting doctors are likewise a diverse group, and battles come in many forms. Once again, the coherence in understandings between patient and physician can be crucial in fostering the value and benefits that accrue from the clinical relationship.

The battle-ready physician can be a boon to certain patients and the metaphor can itself provide therapeutic value. Yet, potent drugs may entail toxic side effects. The physician certainly supports the patient's desire for restoration and health, yet their interests and motivations may diverge. Some persons may accept conservative recommendations for delayed or slowly incremental therapies but may encounter militant physicians who opt for very aggressive interventions. At times, as May points out, for certain commanders every war is a "just war"[39] and whatever can be done should be done. More dramatically, for certain doctors, fighting takes on aesthetic dimensions, and both battles and surgical operations may be described as beautiful notwithstanding the neatly termed "collateral damage from friendly fire." The powerful general, exemplified by certain famous commanders, gains power by becoming untethered from political and civic responsibilities—a tragic model for militant surgeons that spawned the sad observation that the operation was a success, but the patient died; a different and costly form of clinical abdication and failure.

The increasing and valuable role of complex and high technology in medical care may be accompanied by its own set of risks. The highly trained, minimally invasive surgeon, interventional cardiologist, and procedural gastroenterologist may develop a restricted practice dedicated to a narrow array of procedures, all of which entail an increasing distance from the patient. In fact, the surgeon adept at using robotic machines may be many feet removed from the patient, akin to the pilot of a drone thousands of miles from the field of combat. Patients referred to such super-specialists may have been prepared for the procedure by their own physicians so that the person performing the actual intervention may not ever meet the awake patient. Such a patient is both a passive participant and a distant witness to the military encounter between doctor and disease. This is a somewhat extreme example but may be a harbinger of a new technical and contractual clinical relationship in which the "proceduralist" is a skilled and sought-after mercenary, who may enjoy the independence of such fighters from continuing obligations and extended responsibilities and who are also freed from the duty to explain and inform. In a technologized mindset of special expertise in a culture steeped in electronic and mechanical marvels, the opportunity to intervene may become an imperative to do so. This new model promises a reductionist and impersonal form of medical care that may be inappropriate and unacceptable to a community of patients already distressed and angered by a confusing and frightening system of health care. To be sure, there are risks for the militant physician as well as for the patient. Patients will not blame the physician for the disease itself but may be disillusioned and angry with a battling doctor who loses the fight. Perhaps the physician may also suffer the loss, just as generals who surrender do not come home to victory parades.

Fighting Words: The Good, the Bad, and the Ugly

Metaphors of battle speak of victory and success, whether the enemy is disease or sin, as understood from the medieval allegory. Eliminating sin brings purity, and conquering disease leads to health. Active engagement replaces passive victimhood and entails a stance of strength, capacity, and empowerment. For many women who resent being viewed by male colleagues and physicians as quiet and responsive to instructions and admonitions, the fighting image instills courage and self-confidence. The militarized patient is the commander with physicians as officers or, alternatively, is an ally engaged in strategic decisions with the physician leading the troops. In either role, the patient acquires agency and some mode of control that can be an antidote to anger and despair. Rage can be directed at the personified and distanced disease and gloom may be alleviated by the competing demands of searching the Internet, consulting with self-help groups, and paying attention to self-care, exercise, and nutrition. The engaged patient gains clearer meanings from a new narrative for a suddenly strange mode of living, takes on responsibilities for daily tasks, and acquires quotidian structure from scheduled treatments and visits, all framed within a striving to win.

There are several general features that characterize the battle myth that explain its beneficial aspects. According to Hawkins, the myth provides an integrated descriptive frame with an internal coherence and, hence, a dimension of comfort. It organizes the narrative arc that brings together the empowered patient, the various members of the treatment team, the strategic plan for success, and the necessary therapeutic modalities and weaponries. The battle trope provides connectivity to the communal war against cancer or disease more generally and inscribes the individual patient into a camaraderie of warriors facing an existential threat. It thereby dissipates the loneliness and provides natural links to support groups and disease-specific associations of advocates. Lastly, the battle concept analogically roots the individual dealing with a particular problem in the greater historical allegory and psychomachia of good versus evil with its deep cultural resonances.[40]

The battle metaphor and its extensions are powerful rhetorical instruments and may entail harms and risks that warrant special caution on the part of physicians and other caregivers. We have noted the risk of denial that may accompany an overwhelming desire to fight and the prospect of loss can come as a harsh realization. The stronger the hope of success, the more daunting is the progression of disease and the worsening of suffering. A public stance of fighting risks not only the burden of battle but the shame of loss and the guilt for what may be understood retrospectively as unfortunate and irrevocable choices. Constant active engagement spells physical and emotional fatigue for the patient and a concern for the suffering of the family. Paradoxically, successes can be diminished by constant fears of recurrence of disease and tainted by symptoms of post-traumatic stress. Survivors who regard themselves as victors often opt to forget the battle and even avoid reminders of success. The decision to fight can lead to another form of guilt and shame—of not having fought sufficiently hard to win. Family members and physicians may spur a patient to adopt a more martial role than the individual might desire. Indeed, acquiring agency and pride of being in control presumes that the initial choice was a genuine decision and not one imposed by the expectations of others who may be well-intentioned but underestimate the importance of a choice freely made that is then endorsed and supported by family and physicians alike. The fighting stance also mandates the need to maintain an optimistic public persona. Patients can become entrapped in a thumbs-up, brave, and stoic performative identity that can forestall the evolution from battle to acceptance and the development of a means of coping with the different phases of an illness. Hawkins depicts a husband who "rebukes his wife for taking the pain killers she obviously needs and reproaches her for 'giving in.'" Shortly before his wife's death, the husband adds, "if [she] gives in now, both she and I'll lose respect for her ... these are her last days. They're her final chance to show everybody what a fine person she is."[41]

If the battle metaphor is to serve as an integrative, coherent model for a patient, it must be shared by the physician. Or, at the very least, the physician must appreciate the particular framing that best responds to the needs of the person who is ill and adapt the clinical approach to provide the mechanisms and meanings the individual requires. A patient who desires to take charge and mount a campaign against the disease may not be well served by a surgeon who opts for a conservative treatment plan. Such a clinical relationship will be strained unless the doctor understands the differing world views of the patient and invests the time and attention to explain the recommended approach or agrees to work in concert to choose a different though clinically appropriate modality of treatment. Conversely, a methodical, careful patient who prefers to seek many opinions and consider all options may be easily overwhelmed by an assertive and overbearing military medical figure. A more extreme example is a person whose demands for details and careful examination of the many choices now readily accessible via the Internet may irritate the physician. The ensuing battle may indeed be between patient and physician, to the detriment of both parties.

Perhaps the most common mismatch between patient and caregiver stems from the reality that patients' attitudes and stances toward their illnesses and their caregivers may change during their particular clinical trajectories. At the same time, the personas of the physicians remain rather stable, though they may change over the course of a career, a rather different timeline. Patients differ one from another and change with time, thus underlining the imperative for clinicians to be singularly attuned to the great diversity of persons seeking care and the evolution of their attitudes and needs over the span of life and illness.

What then accounts for the longevity and resilience of the war metaphor in medicine in Western society? Part of the answer lies in the deeply engrained origins of the trope in the allegories of good and evil that permeate our narratives and literature. Many of our frames are oppositional and dialectic and the battle concept in the clinic aligns with more general attitudes toward human identity. Our fables and histories speak of battles and conflicts and triumphs over chaos and turmoil. *Homo economicus* strives in a world of winners and losers and our beloved pastimes celebrate victories, whether on the sports field, the casino, or the chessboard. The notion of war in medicine certainly gained energy with the discovery of actual enemies in the guise of bacteria to supplement the more ethereal miasmas and evil influences. Protective vaccination was followed by the discovery of oppositional "anti-bodies" and "anti-biotics" that provided the armamentarium for modern incarnations of the older metaphysical allegories. The clear successes of microbiology and immunology underlined the power of the battle tropes and may also have blinded us to their potent toxicities. It is not surprising to find examples of persons and patients for whom such frames provide comfort and meaning in coping with serious illness. At the same time, our imperative as caregivers is to understand how such tropes do their linguistic, cognitive, and affective work and to remain sensitive and attentive to their often hidden dangers and threats to the welfare of patients in particular and society more generally.

III

FRAMES AND CHOICES

8
In Other Words

Emerson, whose memory failed him in the last years of his life, [had] friends [who] described him not as deteriorating but as living in a protracted state of dreaming. Perhaps here is a better model.... "Dreaming does not necessarily inspire dread; rather, dreaming is considered a part of life, albeit one of its stranger manifestations. Dreamers do not endure social stigma, humiliation or ostracization. To the contrary, dreaming metaphors often invoke tender, even spiritual, qualities."

—"Better Care for Dementia Patients Begins With New Metaphors."
New York Times, April 22, 2020

"I worry that the language we think describes a reality," Lynn Casteel Harper explains, "also creates one."[1] Her concern hinges on the public discourse on dementia that has been dominated by the same tropes used to warn of the impending catastrophic effects of climate change, namely, a looming disaster, a tsunami, and a gray plague. She expresses the fear that these tropes add to the suffering of those with Alzheimer's disease, their caregivers, and everyone else in the at-risk population—"that is, all of us who plan to grow old." This framing generates a sense of dread but falls short of creative solutions other than the cry to arms, "battle amyloid." The exhortation did elicit a strong response by charitable organizations active in the domain of dementia. They invested enormous sums in biological research searching for a causal mechanism in alliance with pharmaceutical firms that sponsored testing efforts to identify persons at risk for dementia, described as "carriers" for an elusive gene for Alzheimer's disease. The drug companies then tested novel interventions to rid the brain of the putatively causal amyloid proteins. In the end, such human carriers were left to live in fear of impending disease when the clinical trials did not lead to any new drugs to prevent the onset or treat the persons at risk or those with overt illness.

While research on causality and therapy are appropriate and necessary, it is also evident that the language of a "gray tsunami" and the "war on Alzheimer's" has engendered dread and fear, and has skewed attitudes toward dementia and the care of persons with this illness. Single-minded attention to aggressive experimental interventions to seek cures for what may be an exaggerated process of aging has obscured other framings and undermined alternative health care initiatives. The enlightenment philosopher Giambattista Vico described metaphors as myths in miniature: we now speak of persons with memory loss as "victims" and those with dementia as having "vanished." The myth of battle is reinforced by what Harper describes as "cultural bigotry against cognitive impairment and old age,"[2] while sufferers are deemed "socially dead." As a result, our expectation of an absolute cure distracts us from a sober consideration of the "realistic 'postponement' of the more debilitating effects of brain aging that can be achieved by modifying known biological, psychosocial, and environmental risk factors."[3] This overweening powerful metaphor blocks us from searching for more benign and perhaps more useful perspectives on the cognitive changes that may accompany old age. Without nuanced figurative language, we cannot describe complex and emotionally laden questions of life nor adequately communicate our responses and needs. To escape the narrow constraints on our thinking, and to avoid the label of "burden" when we think of those with losses of memory or other functional capacities, we need to move beyond military tropes and develop new constellations of words that can change our ways of seeing the world and the people within it.

Reimagining Illnesses through New Language

Biomedical and psychosocial research continually add to our understanding of our bodies and selves both in health and illness. We develop novel theories and gather new data that have the potential to reform what we know and how we think about humans, persons, bodies, and psyches, and the ailments, both old and new, to which we are vulnerable. However, new ideas can reshape our mindsets and imaginations only if couched in novel metaphors and newly minted expressions and framings. New ideas cannot rewire cognitive networks if articulated in old, constraining language. It is through the surprises and awakenings made possible by new linguistic tropes that we apprehend and construct new realities. Furthermore, only new realities—or an appreciation of the illusions of old misunderstandings—permit us to entertain novel thoughts and, in consequence, to enact new behaviors. Language, as the organizer of perceptions into coherent views of the world, is the necessary interpreter that permits us to see the consequences of new information and theories and is the mediator among insights, thoughts, and actions. New tropes can lead to new thoughts and behaviors and effect reshaped understandings of patients and their illnesses. To return to an image we explored earlier: if language is the house of being, then new ways of seeing and living in the world require linguistic renovations.

Insofar as the mediation of words as the shapers of thoughts is a foundational concept in clinical medicine, it is useful to consider additional instances of insights from research that have spurred novel and productive framings of causality and pathogenesis of disease and illness. While we have long known that microorganisms that live within and around us may lead to infections, we now appreciate that, somewhat paradoxically, bacteria in the gut are necessary for the proper functioning of our brains and the regulation of our emotional balance. This expansive appreciation of contextual factors and of the complexity of biological and social networks has led to a contextually and environmentally situated understanding that demands a change in how we talk about human health and illness. Chronic traumatic encephalopathy of professional athletes and others, soldiers in particular, who experience recurrent concussive head injuries is another case in point. The ultimate effects of such trauma are manifest in shrunken brains and impaired cognitive function. This ailment of young men, whether caused on the battlefield or in a sports stadium, is sadly due to controllable social factors. The development of dementia in young and otherwise healthy athletes and soldiers may help us appreciate cognitive decline within a reframed ecological understanding. A different example, not of dementia but susceptibility to a viral infection, comes from the dramatic diversity in illnesses during the COVID-19 pandemic. In metropolitan New York City, rates of infections and mortality varied substantially, with higher rates in the Bronx than in other boroughs. In neighborhoods with the highest COVID-19 infection rates, about a fourth of the residents had college degrees compared to half of residents in those with the lowest rates. These are but a few of the many social determinants that contribute to the health and well-being of a society and its individual members. A person's income, occupation, diet, gender, race, and particular status in the social and economic hierarchies within a country are major factors in determining that individual's morbidity and longevity. These are factors in a personal ecology that in turn interact within the backdrop of a social ecology, namely, the extent of family support, community groups, social cohesion, availability of recreation and games, and opportunities for hobbies and lifelong learning, and the sense of control and agency afforded to persons and groups. Interestingly, it is not necessarily the absolute levels of wealth, education, and social class but rather the extremes of hierarchy and stratification within the society that are the strongest correlates of social, emotional, and physical well-being. Finally, the interconnectedness of the global community provides a third and broader notion of ecology that includes such features as climate change, access to nutrition, endemic diseases, and catastrophic pandemics. In brief, human well-being is dependent on social, economic, and environmental factors, as well as political and cultural factors, that together constitute the social determinants of health.

The introduction of the social determinants of health as factors in pathogenesis of disease and illness can only be accommodated with newer metaphors, in this instance of a human ecology to replace tropes of war and battles. To appreciate how such new framings influence our societal conception of disease, we return to dementia by way of illustration. Daniel George, a medical anthropologist, uses the metaphor of ecology to characterize a school for inner-city students at which "elders with dementia who live at neighboring long-term care homes [are] reading books with children, sharing life history narrative, singing songs, and co-creating crafts."[4] Such persons with memory loss are transformed from victim into mentor and thereby gain a "role in protective local networks that can preserve status, purpose, and quality of life."[5] No longer viewed as abandoned or vanished, such aging persons are "potential contributors rather than merely … an amorphous collective burden."[6] Dementia is no longer a target with "bellicose words like 'prevent', 'halt', 'reverse', 'fight', 'arrest', and 'cure' that promise more than science can deliver, while metaphorically rendering the brain a seat of violence." The ecological metaphor advises "prevention-oriented thinking on diet, exercise, cognitive and social engagement, purpose, and participation in community"[7] as means of delaying the progression of symptoms and improving the quality of life of those who are growing old. A recent review article notes, "The implementation of long-term, multidomain interventions designed for the modification of multiple vascular risk factors and the maintenance of socially-integrated lifestyles and mentally-stimulating activities is expected to postpone the clinical onset of AD [Alzheimer's disease] and dementia."[8] In addition to helping those with dementias, the ecological framing brings benefits to caregivers, families, and communities. As George points out, "a shift away from the metaphors that portray caregiving as a state of constant bereavement may emancipate the full spectrum of emotions felt by caregivers: not just the deep sadness and distress that are intrinsic to the experience, but also the humor, love, compassion, forgiveness, reconciliation, and other sentiments involved in caring for a loved one with dementia. Caring is not only about shouldering day-to-day responsibilities, but is also an opportunity to return kindness and warmth to parents, relatives, or friends in their time of need, and an invitation to slow down and become more introspective in one's own life."[9] We can bring to bear the concepts of personhood, integrity and dignity, prevention, and resilience and a "vernacular of higher ideals and values—as well as new language patterns rising out of the ecological movement."[10]

Traditional Chinese Medicine

A set of metaphors starkly different from the violent tropes of Western societies is evident in East Asian understandings of health and illness. The most commonly cited examples are found in traditional Chinese medicine (TCM) that understands health to consist in appropriate balances of body fluids and other components and their necessary flows along channels or meridians of the body. Aaron Stibbe, a professor of ecological linguistics, has pointed out that military metaphors are rare in contemporary books on TCM and cites as an example a 1991 volume on oncology. At most, a textbook might refer to a "harsh environmental condition"[11] as an enemy. The body is an integrated energetic system and healing entails relieving blocked flows of ch'i along body meridians by acupuncture and other means of restoring harmony. TCM understands the human body in physiological, rather than morphological or anatomic terms, and disease as a state of imbalance, not a reified invading entity.

The introduction of contemporary Western medicine into Chinese medical culture permits a comparison between older and more recent understandings. Illness in traditional medicine is set in the context of the body as a holistic system, whereas Western medicine sees disease as a mechanical breakdown of a machine, with an imperative to repair or replace a specific failing part. Western metaphors of war with their fights and battles have influenced contemporary medical thinking in East Asia, while TCM strives to remain concerned about the elements of nature and the influence of weather and food on the emergence and treatment of illness. These are then two competing systems with very different conceptions of illness and healing.

Jing Bao Nie and colleagues reviewed the metaphors used to characterize HIV-related illnesses following the advent of antiretroviral therapies and describe a shift from fighting and curing to living with the disease. They describe an evolution in thinking from a state of war to a perpetual truce. In their analysis, the authors allude to a form of modified or transformed military metaphors that they find in eighteenth-century TCM. They note that when TCM uses military language, the aim is prevention, not intervention after the fact. TCM tells us that "in the golden days of old the sages did not treat the disease after it had already set in but before it began."[12] Moreover, the hierarchy in TCM assigns to the patient the role of sovereign while the physician is the general, while quickly noting that the five cardinal virtues of a military general were "wisdom, sincerity, humaneness, courage and strictness"[13] and "the supreme principal of war is to win without fighting." Thus, the meaning of military metaphors used in an East Asian cultural context is transformed so that they do not bear the entailments of all-out battle to the end. Rather, they connote optimistic and positive meanings of "balance, prevention, peace, pacification and humaneness."[14]

TCM is an instructive amalgam of constructs reminiscent of ancient Western humoral theories of Greek medicine, with its balances of natural forces, and of recent tropes in Western medicine and culture that foreground ecological sensibilities with attention to the local and global environments in which people develop and live.

Ecological Metaphors

Natural and ecological figures in East Asian traditions are evident in certain indigenous societies in sub-Saharan Africa. Lives in such settings are experienced in communities that include people, animals, and spirits. Nature is ever-present: living means coexistence with both animate and inanimate forces, and domination of nature is not in the realm of possibilities. Illnesses are accepted as natural and inevitable and phenomena that one cannot exterminate. While illness cannot be fought or overpowered, nonetheless, one may yet cope with misfortune with treatments that "coax and plead with the illness to leave its innocent victim alone."[15]

George Annas, a legal scholar and bioethicist, cites the aphorism of the writer William S. Burroughs, "Language is a virus,"[16] to underline the potency of language in spreading its influence. He opines in an article in the *New England Journal of Medicine* that restructuring the American health care system necessitates replacing the traditional military and newer market metaphors that can no longer serve as leitmotifs to care. He turns to the ecology movement as a source for relevant words, such as "integrity," "balance," "natural," "limited (resources)," "quality (of life)," "diversity," "renewable," "sustainable," "responsibility (for future generations)," "community," and "conservation." While his prescription is for the health care system on a national if not global scale, he points to the value of an ecological trope for individual lives, both healthy and ill. Annas emphasizes that "the ecologic metaphor could, for example, help us confront and accept limits (both on expectations about the length of our lives and on the expenditure of resources we think reasonable to increase longevity), to value nature, and emphasize the quality of life. This metaphor could lead us to worry about our grandchildren, and thus plan for the long term, to favor sustainable technology over technology we cannot afford to provide to all who could benefit from it, to emphasize prevention and public health measures, and to debate the merits of rationing."[17] He notes the implications of ecological thinking in demanding attention to the social determinants of health and to enhanced efforts at prevention, a long-neglected poor relation. Such reframing has the potential to moderate our long-standing enchantment with high technology in medicine and the rights of individuals and draw attention to communitarian ideas of healthy living and the duties of all citizens.

In the aftermath of a global pandemic, the concept of ecology reminds us once again that humans cannot be separated from nature and the life forms among which we live. Risk of mortality during the most recent plague was linked to the chronic illnesses of lifestyles and our own choices, both individual and societal. While the language of war has been an ever-present trope in our collective responses to epidemics, the ecological metaphors may in fact be more helpful in teaching us what went wrong and how to best prevent a recrudescence of disease and a return to crisis. Indeed, our best means of diminishing impact are our own behaviors in a thoroughly ecological framework of prudent isolation, self-care, handwashing, and an attitude of optimistic patience. New language couched in ecological terms may finally reshape our tropes and our thoughts and, thereby, our behaviors.

Balance and Homeostasis

The concept of homeostasis was developed and promulgated by Walter Cannon at Harvard in the 1930s to characterize the physiological systems of the body that regulate and maintain within strict limits many important parameters relevant to survival and health. Thus, for example, blood sugar, pH, body temperature, serum electrolytes, and many similar body conditions are kept in a state of balance or equilibrium, and the term *homeostasis* became a guiding metaphor for physiologists and physicians for almost a century. In turn, disease could be envisaged as a loss of equilibrium or a condition of "dystasis" that demands medical attention to ameliorate and correct the state of imbalance. The idea of equilibrium was further elaborated by French physician and philosopher Georges Canguilhem, who notes that "nature, within man as well as without, is harmony and equilibrium. The disturbance of this harmony, this equilibrium, is called disease."[18] The idea of balance and harmony are consonant with the East Asian models of flow and equilibrium of yin and yang, as well as with ecological concepts of the internal milieu and the environmental conditions of the natural world. Understood in this context, disease is a process, not a reified entity to be fought. Canguilhem notes that "disease … for the sick man … [is] really another way of life."[19] The patient's experience of illness is all-encompassing and the sufferer, not simply the laboratory data and the computer images, demands attention. The clinician's mandate is to assist nature in the restoration of the person to the antecedent or, more often, to a new state of equilibrium. Canguilhem's definition of disease as that of the sick man, not that of the doctor, effectively underwrites a truly patient-oriented medicine. The ill person gains agency and control without the negative consequence of losing, since the imperative is not that of winning, but rather restoration to a state of health extant prior to the illness or, at least, to a situation of sustained peaceful coexistence. Restoration is measured in functional capacities and the patient is the arbiter of that state of being and the adequacy of the new equilibrium to the goals of the individual's continuing existence and life.

The distinction between the state prior to illness and a new equilibrium point acknowledges the reality of human biology and illness: healing is common; curing in the sense of complete return to an Edenic state of purity is rare. To return to a previous example, antiretroviral therapy permits persons with HIV to return to a full and long life, albeit in a perpetual equilibrium with what may be a latent virus. A person who has suffered a stroke may, with modifications to the home and place of work, return to a prior experience of life, work, and family. The person no longer feels ill even though the physician can measure the permanent remnants of neurological loss. While it is the case that the person may not be able to return to a previous level of skill at tennis or golf, the individual can, with human resilience in concert with supportive clinicians, adapt to new and adequate set points of balance. This is what is meant by restoration to a new equilibrium with a new fulcrum point that sustains a regained sense of harmony. This metaphoric alternative is at once optimistic and provides agency and control. Canguilhem underlines this capacity of resilience and asserts that "the healthy state [is] much more than the normal state. It is the state which allows transitions to new norms."[20] Indeed, the ability to reimagine a new normal may be the true goal of the person who is ill and who desires to attain a "state of health [that] is a state of unawareness where the subject and the body are one."[21] The ideal recovery is to be capable of forgetting the prior illness and suffering. This objective may be a more realistic and attainable conception of health than a state of innocence.

Illness as Journey

Narratives of journeys, both actual and metaphoric, are universal. Stories of discovery of exotic as well as inner spaces, time travel, *Bildungsromane*, spiritual quests, and tales of pilgrimages are a celebrated genre of poetry and prose. The trope of a journey is often found in stories of illness and is an important species of pathography, whether by patients or their families. In her study of pathographies, Anne Hawkins notes that journey and battle myths are the most common tropes in the stories that patients construct to make sense of their illnesses. The journey involves travel to a different world that is "surprising, terrible, wonderful." The travelers to the "kingdom of the sick" make sense of the new rituals they encounter as patients and draw on "archaic connotations of heroism and courage" that may restore feelings of "personal dignity and social value."[22] Oliver Sacks, describing his recovery from a leg injury, relies on the image of a pilgrimage and "a journey of the soul" through a state of "limbo" and "the dark night of the soul."[23] The feelings of strangeness and exile described by patients lead Hawkins to recall the phenomenon of liminality used by the anthropologist Victor Turner to describe the rites of passage evident in many societies. These include ceremonies of coming-of-age, initiation into privileged clubs and societies, and rituals of installation and cycles of life. These rites are often characterized by three phases: separation from the ordinariness of daily life, a liminal phase of alienation lasting days or weeks, and finally reincorporation into a new status in society. This view of the journey of illness, perhaps with a hospital stay for serious illness, reflects the "passivity, humility, and near-nakedness"[24] that characterize the liminality of patienthood. The return, with its promise of re-aggregation into family and society, perhaps with a new and longed-for status of health, is the optimistic and hoped-for conclusion. For many, the period of isolation provides a quiet space for reflection and a realization that the recovery must be to a new state of balance. As Virginia Woolf writes in her essay "On Being Ill," for the person who is ill, "the world has changed its shape; the tools of business grown remote; the sounds of festival ... heard across far fields."[25] For those who are fortunate to return to health, the new state of being is replete with new meanings and perhaps with reshaped identities.

The metaphor of journey is distinct from the better known military frame. A journey avoids the adversarial stance while providing a sense of purpose and direction. A trip entails decisions about destination and route and affords a sense of agency and control while avoiding the specter of loss on a foreign field of war. The patient has a variety of options that can be empowering—one may choose the role of driver of the bus with the physician as navigator or simply opt to be a passenger and a more passive traveler. In either case, the patient is offered the opportunity of choosing a role consonant with that individual's persona and outlook. Persons who are members of common patient interest groups or those receiving care in the same treatment center can become traveling companions, thus diminishing the sense of isolation and loneliness experienced by many with serious illnesses. The arc of time shifts from a static waiting for something to happen to moving toward a desired milestone or, ideally, return from a successful pilgrimage. A journey permits layovers and rest stops and time for respite and recuperation. There is a road map and less fear of what lies ahead; travel is not inherently confrontational and rarely disastrous. Perhaps, most significantly, if the journey does not end well, there is no attribution of guilt or blame for having lost a fight.

Reisfield notes that the journey metaphor is increasingly apt in the domain of oncology as rates and lengths of survival increase steadily. Cancer "has largely been transformed from an acute event to a chronic illness, enmeshed in life narratives that may span years or even decades.... [T]he journey metaphor ... allows for discussions of goals, direction, and progress.... [It] has the depth, richness, and gravitas to be applicable to the cancer experience."[26] The comment that serious illness requires metaphors with "gravitas" and language that must show thoughtfulness and respect is a worthy lesson for clinicians. A further benefit to a journey is the shift of mindset for many patients who have felt themselves in their premorbid daily lives traveling "on cruise control, often at high-speed." As patients, they can now "exit the freeway" and embark on a quieter journey that permits "the discovery of new sources of meaning; wells of courage, strength, and determination"[27] and a renewed sense of self. Many patients describe a newfound sense of humility and gratitude gained on their journeys of discovery.

A similar instance of the journey trope is provided by Nie, with a description of HIV disease in Africa. Now that this illness is a chronic condition, a common description of a diagnosis is a "bus ticket" and "waiting to board" with hope for a "long journey."[28] The trip may be lifelong and while there may be "unexpected turn[s]" the perspective is directed to the future and new opportunities "on the road to a cure."[29]

For too many others faced with life-threatening illness, the journey is hardly that of the tourist or happy wanderer. The travel unfolds in uncharted territory and the exploration of the unknown may be dark and threatening. Here the value of the journey metaphor, according to Reisfield, is that it "does not countenance such concepts as winning, losing, and failing. Rather, there are only different roads to travel, various avenues to be explored, and, always, there are exits." However, he cautions us to be aware that "the roads may be bumpy and poorly illuminated at times, and one may encounter forks, crossroads, roadblocks, U-turns, and detours."[30] Uncertainty of what lies beyond a curve remains and the journey may end all too soon. Semino and colleagues assessed the use of journey metaphors in the online writings of patients and discovered examples of both "empowering" and "disempowering"[31] language. In the former category they place patients with non-adversarial roles taking charge of journeys and the presence of traveling companions. By contrast, rides may be wild or roller-coaster with many ups and downs as well as twists and turns. Journeys may end up in the wilderness and the patient at the wheel may with time become a reluctant traveler. Perrault and O'Keefe find that patients may fear a "trainwreck" that may ensue from a "runaway train ... going downhill"[32] and "a yellow brick road fraught with pain, danger and loss."[33] They cite the author Jenny Diski, who writes both about travel and her own time as a patient with breast cancer and observes that while "journeys ... have become coupled with optimism," they are susceptible to calamities and may "not end well or in the right place." More optimistically, however, journeys "engage emotions associated not with division and conflict, but with movement and connection between people."[34]

The journey metaphor can provide a less burdensome opportunity for living with, rather than fighting, illness. There are two major considerations or caveats that clinicians must keep in mind so that their patients reap benefits from this approach. First, the patient must be enabled and indeed supported in choosing the specific metaphor to narrate the illness. That is, the choice must resonate with the particular person's mindset and identity and must be free of any coercion. Second, the journey must engage the physician as guide, supporter, and companion on the journey. Some patients will prefer to steer the bus, others will choose to navigate, while there are those who will wish to be guided once the direction and destination have been chosen in tandem with the treating clinician. Patients should not feel they have been sent on a journey alone, and certainly not abandoned to the vagaries of the currents and the winds. Yet, somewhat surprisingly, pathographies rarely describe physicians as guides on the journey. Hawkins cites one author who explains that "the failure to provide safe conduct is the most serious shortcoming in cancer treatment today."[35] She notes that physicians find it easier to be generals than guides, resulting in both a failure to listen and a failure of care. Journeys become isolating and frightening when unguided and thus fail to provide the needed sense of security, optimism, and hope. Rather than providing comfort, a journey unaccompanied by the physician may be experienced as abandonment, when what is desired and required are guidance and attentiveness. Reisfield and Wilson underline these responsibilities, stating that "physicians may be trusted and knowledgeable guides, accompanying the patient throughout the journey, one that may ultimately imbue them both with a vision of a deeper meaning in life."[36] Penson and colleagues expand on these clinical imperatives by adding, "I am looking for metaphors that help me let that patient know I acknowledge where they are, I can bear it with them, and maybe I can offer them some perspective."[37] And, "through language the doctor needs to provide mile markers in the patient's journey, to tell the patient roughly where they are, and to signal them when there is a drastic change.... [T]he language that we use puts patients onto some path of recovery, helps them cope.... I think our language can be enormously powerful in helping patients understand the disease trajectory and moments of transition."[38] As for children who are ill, these authors prefer the metaphor of work and getting a job done together, by clinician and child. The child must not be left to believe that the task is a sole responsibility, lest failure is construed as bearing blame and guilt. The needed clinical skills of language demand thoughtfulness and learning. Anatole Broyard reminds us that "astute as he is, [the young physician] doesn't yet understand that all cures are partly 'talking cures.' Every patient needs mouth-to-mouth resuscitation, for talk is the kiss of life."[39]

The Quest Narrative

In his work on the stories of illness, the sociologist Arthur Frank describes three basic narratives that patients use to make meaning of their lives through the experience of severe illness. The restitution narrative is a tale of illness and recovery. It is the most desired and certainly the most optimistic and a good story as it speaks in retrospect about cure and restoration to health. In stark contrast, the chaos story describes severe illness with a sense of darkness and fear. Difficulties in ascertaining a clear diagnosis are compounded by bureaucratic incompetence to result in a hopeless breakdown of normal existence. It is a tale of suffering, and its sense of hopelessness threatens the healthy listener. The third type, and of specific interest to the notion of journeys, is the narrative of quest.

The quest narrative is the tale of a traveler who has experienced a chronic illness and a long voyage. It is neither triumphant nor dark, but neither is its denouement that of cure and happy recovery. The quest story tells of a journey of experience and learning. It often reflects a quiet and humble gratitude for lessons learned and insights gained on the road that were, paradoxically, made possible by illness. Quest stories tell of self-discovery as a consequence of illness and an unanticipated gift. "Quest stories are about illness leading to new insights."[40] New ways of being and living are discovered with new friendships and unexpected identities. The quest narrative is replete with experiences to be shared and taught and resonates not with joy but with "wisdom."[41] Thus, something of value is "reclaimed" from the journey and what has been gained gives structure to the story and perhaps meaning to the life as lived. The narrators of these stories of quests are "ancient mariners,"[42] who "look not to restitution but rather to what can be reclaimed of life: what can be learned, and how this lesson can be passed on to those who have not made their journey."[43]

The quest narrative brings its own challenges and caveats. A quest implies abandoning the goals of restitution and cure. It means giving up victory for the realistic and tangible benefit of discovering a new self. Frank cites a patient who reports, "Deep illness requires giving up the old self, the person you used to be" and advises other patients to "find your way to be somebody else, the next viable you."[44] Frank cautions us to remember that quest narratives may be witnessed as "subversive" by listeners. Physicians, not surprisingly, prefer stories of cures and happy outcomes and may resist other constructions of illness and the added burdens on them that these may entail—not least the imperative of listening to the patient. Family members may continue to seek the healthy persona of their loved one who is ill and resist the implicit declaration that restitution is no longer an option. Thus, "quest stories are about being forced to accept life unconditionally,"[45] and perhaps only patients are capable of gratitude for a reclaimed life, however long or short.

Missing Metaphors

Viruses have become an important concern of global public health and at the same time have burgeoned over the past quarter-century as a metaphor for diverse aspects of our culture. Many computer users run applications to cleanse their hard drives of contaminating viruses that arrive as Trojan horses accompanying malware. The hyperlinked world of the Web and data networks has spawned viral memes that disseminate information like global infections and viral spread is en route to becoming a ubiquitous and perhaps embedded trope. As we have noted previously, language itself has been compared to a virus. Not least, we witness the excitement in the media when an alluring idea or striking fashion fad goes viral.

And yet, when the virus named corona is not at all metaphoric but all too real, we fall back on our ancient and burnished military tropes that have, one might say, gone viral during the pandemic. We have declared war, health care workers are heroes on the frontlines, politicians demand strategies from war cabinets, and our new armor are gowns, gloves, masks, and ventilators. It is more than passing strange that we are asked to fight with inactivity, by retreating to our homes and lying low till some unknown future permits us to venture forth once again. This efflorescence of battle rhetoric has in many countries clouded the actual need for management by screening and contact tracing and led to the unfortunate use of unproven toxic medications. The imperative to fight the unseen has stimulated fear and uncertainty with an emerging toll of mental illness. It has shifted attention away from the need for continuing daily care for urgent medical conditions and interrupted long-standing programs of routine preventive vaccinations of infants and children. Perhaps more egregiously, the desire for herd immunity has made palatable the idea of collateral damage and inured us to scandalous mortality rates in homes for the elderly and infirm.

The imperative to fight blinds us to the social conditions that enable the spread of the virus—namely, poverty, crowding, malnutrition, and dramatic disparities of income and social opportunities. Concurrently, the presumed battles against the disease have been paralleled by bitter political rivalries with recommendations shaped not by data sets and evidence but by sociopolitical ideologies. We have failed to search for and employ alternative tropes to replace the military metaphors decried by many health care providers and commentators. We sorely need metaphors and conceptual frameworks that engender compassion and support, stimulate clear and consistent communication and information, provide a sense of cautious optimism, begin to acknowledge deep-seated social inequities, and permit the collaborations, both locally and internationally, that can lead to a broad consensus on pathways through the complexities of the current turmoil and that concurrently shape a different and better post-pandemic world. To do so, however, we will also need to find the appropriate tropes to enlighten the journeys.

Figures of Speech

The varieties of human experience and diversity of illnesses indicate that a broad array of tropes are needed to permit individuals to frame and make sense of their particular, unique lives as patients. The military metaphor is best known and widely encountered, and concepts of flow, balance, journey, and sports are alternatives chosen by many. Some patients opt for less common metaphors that emanate from life experiences. One patient brought to bear a "building project as a metaphor for his cancer treatment. He developed a set of metaphoric correspondences (e.g., setbacks such as radiation burns or neutropenia were 'change orders' or 'delays in the project') that helped him organize and communicate his cancer experience."[46] Others prefer mountaineering, a chess match, a dramatic performance, or simply a job to be done.

Underlying this series of different mindsets are common elements that caregivers must respect and affirm. First, metaphors are valuable in understanding and coping with the unexpected interruptions of life by illness. Whether the need is to understand mysterious causalities, choose therapies, or adapt to new circumstances, language may help or harm, but will always be required. Even the light-hearted description by a mother of a routine visit with infant to a pediatrician as a "five-thousand-mile checkup and oil change" helps place the need for preventive health care into the ordinariness of daily chores. Metaphors are ubiquitous, and sensitivity to their use by patients and families is a necessary clinical skill.

Second, the value of the metaphor to a given person depends on many idiosyncratic aspects of background, experiences, mindset, attitudes, and values—a complex mélange whose details may be difficult to decipher. It is only through specific attention and careful listening to how a person tells and constructs the story of illness and the personal reactions to the uncertainty and fear that a physician can appreciate which tropes are appropriate and relevant to that person and context. Then, as Perrault and O'Keefe note, "care providers can tune their use of the metaphor to each person's understanding of what it means."[47] Imposition of a caregiver's own particular choice on a patient is inappropriate, in the same fashion that insisting on a particular therapy with which a patient expresses concern or discomfort is wrong. That is not to say that thoughtful advice and guidance should be withheld. A thoughtful clinician who understands that a successful outcome of recovery and restitution is unlikely for a certain patient must tread the fine line of avoiding false reassurance without shattering a sense of hope and belief. This onerous clinical task necessitates a high degree of patience bolstered by deep listening and compassion. While metaphors are necessarily shaped by and for the patient, they may change with the course of illness and the goals of care. Once again, this demands a certain vigilance from the clinician, who must adapt to the evolving needs and desires of the patient. At times, these shifts may be subtle and nuanced and require careful probing and compassionate inquiry. Lastly, and perhaps most important, is to recall the obligation of the clinician to serve as both guide and, as needed, companion in care and caring. The patient may find comfort in tropes of war, sports, journeys, or quests and must be supported in these sources of personal meaning. The clinician must find the means of expression and the modalities of language to remain present to the patient, whatever the outcome.

9
Listening

When the physician is truly present and open to hear, the patient will be more fully present and able to speak.

—Michael Balint

A story needs a listener. I needed their gift of listening in order to make my suffering a relationship between us, instead of an iron cage around me.

—Arthur Frank

In our everyday lives, we value communication and appreciate the importance of human interactions, both verbal and nonverbal. There is a moment to speak and a time to listen, and we generally presume these actions are reciprocal and balanced. Similarly, it appears self-evident that words and conversations are necessary to clinical interactions among colleagues and crucial to encounters between patients and their physicians. And yet, the physician's failure to listen is among the most common complaints from patients, and research studies attest to their experiences. An analysis of over one hundred carefully documented clinic visits at a major medical center revealed that the patient's concern or reason for the visit was elicited in only a third of these clinical encounters. Furthermore, when appropriate questions were actually posed, patients' responses were interrupted seven out of ten times, generally after not more than eleven seconds.[1]

To develop an inventory of the attributes of excellent physicians, Donald Boudreau and colleagues asked patients and their families to identify the characteristics of good doctors.[2] They discovered that all fifty-eight persons they interviewed talked about the physician's listening skills and considered those skills of prime importance for them and their families. One patient noted that a capacity to listen was an essential feature of a good doctor and another described this trait as "être à l'écoute"—being in a state of listening. When probed for the reasons for the importance of listening, not surprisingly, many pointed to gathering information for diagnosis. Several noted the therapeutic benefits of listening, including the calming effect of the interaction and, more poignantly, as one patient stated, "if you listen to the patient [you] give the patient respect."[3]

How can we understand why listening by physicians is a sine qua non for clinical care and underscored by patients reflecting on their experiences, yet is found deficient in studies of seemingly well-intentioned doctors working in esteemed centers of health care? Curricula for training health care professionals include courses in communication skills and person-centered care, yet patients continue to express disappointment with terse visits, abrupt questions, and brusque attention from caregivers.

A cursory search of the biomedical literature provides the first inkling of the apparent indifference to listening compared to speaking. The Web of Science database provides access to a vast array of publications in high-quality academic journals from the broad field of science. A search for articles using the expanded search terms for "patient and speak" yielded over 15,000 results. By comparison, a search for "patient and listen" resulted in fewer than 7,000 hits. Moreover, many articles in the latter search were relevant to the field of otolaryngology, that is, physical problems with ears and hearing, rather than listening as an interactive behavior. This differential between speaking and listening is also noted in results of searches in the Medline database of biomedical literature and is more germane to medicine. Here, too, there are twice as many articles about speaking than those dedicated to listening. Of specific interest to medical educators is that of the almost 20,000 papers in the Medline database that deal with teaching, fewer than 200 have as their focus the teaching of listening skills.

The inordinate emphasis on speaking compared with listening is not confined to scientific and biomedical literature, nor are lapses of attention and listening evident only in the hospital and clinic. More generally, speaking is privileged and celebrated in Western culture. Secondary schools offer courses on rhetoric, award prizes for contests in public speaking, and support debating societies. Curricula on persuasive argumentation and rhetorical skills are ubiquitous while course offerings on attentive listening are a rare find. We consider skillful presentations, especially to groups, large and small, as an attribute of leadership and a desirable quality. Speaking is, after all, virile and active; it attracts attention and perhaps even envy. Health care professionals, among others, are expected to explain and clarify difficult and complex notions for their patients and are understandably celebrated for their skills. Articulate exposition has become a surrogate for clinical presence.

By contrast, listening is misunderstood as passive and not requiring any particular skills. Speakers stand out from the crowd—listeners blend in. Listening is not appreciated as challenging or a capacity that can be taught and learned. While a student may understandably express anxiety about an upcoming clinical case presentation, similar fears about an ability to listen properly would strike us as strange.

Listening is second to speaking in our cultural hierarchy, and hearing ranks second to seeing as a sensory modality. We value eyewitness testimony yet mistrust hearsay evidence. Research shows that jurors tend to be more skeptical of hearsay testimony than they are of eyewitness testimony, even though both modalities have been shown to be fallible and prone to faulty recollections.[4] Vision is the root metaphor for thought and in Greek, "to live" is synonymous with "to behold light." Seeing is believing and enlightenment points to understanding. "I saw for myself" and "I see what you mean" are common metaphoric idioms, whereas "I hear you" may introduce a point of disagreement and is often followed by a "But ..." The sense of sight is considered to be reliable; Aristotle judged vision as the sensory modality valued above all others. Yet, he also noted that "for developing thought hearing incidentally takes precedence."[5]

We spend 70 percent of our waking time in communication, with a third of that time engaged in speaking and about half the time listening. Although hearing is our earliest sensory modality and the most common communication tool in daily living, our skills at listening are taken for granted and not understood as a topic for explicit training and development. The social context has contributed to the asymmetry of speaking and listening. We experience an increasing compression of time and the social metronome beats ever more quickly. Long, expository letters that elicited carefully crafted responses gave way to faxed missives that demanded a rapid response, and those in turn have been supplanted by emails with peremptory expectations of rapid decisions and terse answers. Social media have sped up the process of transmission but they are modalities of exposition rather than dialogue. Most messages on social networks are rhetorical, announcing and disseminating bits of information about the sender, rarely anticipating answers other than likes or graphic emoji reactions. Current means of social and cultural communication are all about speaking and have made listening irrelevant. Messages are necessarily short, often set in all-caps, and often ambiguous. However, their nature is consonant with truncated units of time and monologic communication. The Yiddish word for email is *blitzpost*, whose literal rendering is "lightning mail"—a sudden strike from afar that does not anticipate a reasoned response! The paradoxical effect of social media that are celebrated for fostering interactions and connectivities among people is the enhancement of unidirectional speech that neither needs nor fosters dialogue. The already existing constraints on time and space for human interactions are evident in the nature of social media that are further limited by a technology that demands short messages and spawns legions of fuzzy acronyms.

These new technologies have produced a high-speed, interconnected world that is beset by a concurrent degradation of civil discourse. We speak at and past each other, convinced of the truth of our own words and the righteousness of our stances. The plethora of channels of connections has resulted not in more productive talk across boundaries, whether social or disciplinary, but rather in narrow pipelines of unidirectional flow whose messages confirm our truths yet rarely challenge our assumptions. We now live and work in a world that is electronically interconnected yet socially distanced. We suffer the loss of ties that bind, both familial and social, and we are increasingly segregated in silos laced with interconnecting wires but short-circuited communication.

The now ubiquitous electronic health record instantaneously gathers laboratory data, imaging results, and prescription information yet fails to accommodate the words of the physician and the patient, even as it deflects the attention of the doctor from the patient to the computer screen. These systems aid in the seamless flow of clinical data yet paradoxically undermine the continuity of clinical care by easing the interchangeability of caregivers from one clinic visit to the next. The connections that ought to bind patients and physicians are severed, and new relationships must be repeatedly initiated in brief spaces of clinic time. The word *personal* has shifted from a descriptor of an attentive caregiver engaged with a patient and family over a span of years and decades to "personalized" medicine: electronic files replete with idiosyncratic data and numbers intended as descriptive of the given individual. A DNA sequence is now the unique index of the organism and a surrogate for the living person.

The Listening Spectrum

We utilize many different modes of listening in our social interactions. The most common mode of listening in academic circles is the critical style. Many forms of education inculcate a skeptical approach to knowledge and beliefs that may be appropriate in philosophical and intellectual debates and learning. In such settings, careful thinking is construed as a critical attitude. However, when debates shift from an intent to jointly arrive at clarity and consensus to a competitive and even adversarial exercise, then the listener begins with an opening attitude of doubt and skepticism regarding the words of the speaker. The immediate intent is to challenge claims, dispute propositions, and develop counterarguments.

A mutual stance that both interlocutors may be equally right or wrong and the outcome can be a shared belief or, perhaps, a grounded and respectful disagreement is thoroughly dialogic. In this Socratic form of engagement, both listener and speaker desire to learn. By contrast, a doubtful listener who anticipates and is attuned to errors with the goal of winning arguments cannot learn but is open only to confirmation of prior beliefs. This form of unhealthy skepticism is all too common in academic and political debates in which neither party is actually listening and/or able to understand positions with which it disagrees, leading to a pernicious form of confirmation bias and social deafness. Should the speaker detect the arrogance of the critical listener, the words and thoughts may be squelched at the outset, resulting in a stillborn communication. The overall process has been rightly described as critical warfare and hardly as friendly disagreement, whether intellectual or political.

A second form is pseudo-listening. The hearer has little interest in the words of the speaker and is simply waiting, perhaps impatiently, for a turn to speak or a convenient pause to interrupt. While both parties are simply taking turns, there is no dialogue and the thoughts of neither person are shaped by the words of the other. It becomes a dance of two locutors rather than interlocutors, no listeners and hence no learning. Perhaps even no respect. This mode has the benefit of peace unless the interruptions become irritants and there is little warfare as there are no disagreements, only indifference. A variant of pseudo-listening can be observed in group settings, especially when there is a known order of speakers. The individual who has just spoken is busy reflecting on how the words were received and is not attending to the current speaker. The one next in line to speak is also not listening but rather considering the choice of words to follow. In this orderly fashion, a group of six to ten speakers can have the satisfaction of speaking with little risk of being engaged by a thoughtful listener.

Interrogative listening is a complex form with subtypes, each with a hidden agenda. Truly curious questions are genuinely designed to explore the speaker's perspective and expand mutual horizons. By contrast, questions that begin with "Don't you agree …?" or "Wouldn't you say … ?" point to a hidden rhetorical intent to persuade and convince rather than a desire to learn. A second hidden mode is the social probe or judgmental form of questioning whose aim is to discern social status and, one might say, to assess social rather than intellectual capital. The aim of such inquiry is social taxonomy with assignment of individuals to convenient categories. Different forms can be observed during fieldwork, at cocktail parties, and academic gatherings at which competitive jousting is a form of social combat. Both the rhetorical and judgmental subtypes are solipsistic in nature rather than dialogic in spirit. One minor subcategory is listening for record-keeping, designed to amass gossip and build a reserve of socially useful ammunition for later deployment. While this subtype exhibits genuine curiosity, it can hardly be described as generous or respectful. Defensive listening rounds out the array of listening types with self-centered aims—a person who may harbor guilt of some malfeasance or breach and stands ready to rebut any real or perceived accusations. These may be as simple as a mischievous child or as serious as a defendant in a courtroom.

The listening spectrum is broad and can range from full belief to full doubt. There are certainly situations in which the extremes may be appropriate. For example, the listener on a suicide hotline may need to provide a clear sense of complete belief in the gravity of the situation to the distraught caller. A stance of full doubt describes the attitude of a cross-examining barrister in the courtroom. The context, role, and mandate of the listener are all relevant to interactions with the speaker.

Clinical Listening

Listening in the clinic comes in many forms, each appropriate to the moment, context, and purpose. Informational listening by a physician assesses the concerns of the person and the reasons for seeking medical care. More formally, this is the process of taking a medical history so that the clinician may know what to think, that is, to formulate an initial impression of the patient's ailment. These interactions, critical to the mandate of the physician and the goal of attending to the needs of the patient, may be undermined by unhelpful, albeit well-intentioned, habits of many clinicians. Patients experience interruptions sometimes caused by the doctor's eagerness to shorten the visit, even though hasty questions breach the continuity of the patient's narrative and may actually increase the time needed for the interaction to achieve its goal. At times, as is evident also in nonmedical settings, persons who are highly knowledgeable may presume they can predict the information about to be provided and will interrupt the speaker with an intemperate comment, abrogating the full narrative the patient wishes to share. Such interventions may occur early in the course of an interview and lead to inaccurate convictions that in turn become the basis for an anchoring bias.

Even if the early conclusion by the listener does not lead to an overt interruption, the mediating unspoken thought of the listener interferes with that individual's appreciation of the flow of the narrative and may result in the diagnostic error of premature closure, in which a quick initial impression undercuts an openness to countervailing facts, details, and possibilities.

Interruptions by physicians of patients' stories are well documented in the medical literature and are certainly a source of chagrin for patients. Informational listening is central to the acquisition of data and impressions necessary to an accurate diagnosis and to knowing what to think. Haste and interruptions within seconds of the beginning of the patient's rendition lead to inappropriate outcomes and to a lost opportunity for both the narrator and the listener.

A second form of listening in the clinic can be described as transactional and permits the caregiver to "know what I must do." This form is very goal-oriented and instrumental and most often observed in emergency rooms and other acute care settings. Faced with a patient with severe, recent-onset abdominal pain, the surgeon or ICU physician must decide whether a rapid intervention, for example, surgery for a ruptured appendix, is urgently required or a patient with a stroke needs thrombolytic (clot-busting) treatment. In these settings, the listener is closely attuned to the immediate words and behaviors of the patient and is laser-focused on information relevant to a rapid decision. In such instances, close attention is also mandatory, though interruptions may be appropriate if a patient's responses are slow in providing crucial details. Nonetheless, haste that leads to a rapid but incorrect assessment is fraught with great risks of poor outcomes: the imperative of speed must be carefully balanced with the need for accurate decisions. In this context, careful, albeit instrumental, listening is crucial to the tasks at hand and to the quick implementation of care.

Informational and transactional modes of clinical listening have short-term, focused objectives. By contrast, the aims of relational listening, the most important type of clinical listening, are extended in time, deeper in the imperative of engagement, and fundamental to the goals of medicine—namely, the establishment of a therapeutic alliance between patient and physician. Relational listening permits the caregiver to "know who you are and what I must therefore be."

Non-intimate relational listening characterizes outstanding pedagogy that attends to the words, gestures, and expressions of individual students as they learn by speaking to a committed listener. Pastoral care demands sympathetic relational listening to discern subtexts and cryptic meanings in order to identify sources of suffering and angst. The psychiatric stance in medicine is akin to the listening ear of the priest in the confessional. While the mandate and desire to bring relief and assuage spiritual pain are in their own sense instrumental, the capacity to heal necessarily works through the relationship crafted by careful listening and the trust it affords. These interactions are individual, personal though non-intimate, and demand respect for boundaries while respecting confidences. By contrast, relational listening described as intimate refers to highly personal, perhaps romantic, engagements between two persons, generally with complementary vulnerabilities and capacities who have willingly chosen to share deep confidences and intimacies, all fostered by respectful relational listening that is far more than instrumental and intended to create and maintain a deep and evolving dyadic relationship.

Clinical relational listening is both intimate and personal in nature in that confidential information may be revealed together with deeply held and protected fears, doubts, and anxieties. Medical histories and examinations are intimate in character in assessing physical, emotional, social, and mental states. However, the nature of the intimacy is very different from the dyadic/romantic form. In the clinical setting, the two individuals are rather different in vulnerabilities and responsibilities. The patient's bodily integrity may be weakened by illness and the assessment of the world may be clouded by pain, fear, and altered mentation. The interaction is not between equally capable and empowered persons, and this difference in independent agency adds greatly to the responsibilities and duties of the caregiver and the rights of the patient to receive care and attention. The demanding fiduciary obligations of physicians to their patients as described in legal doctrines and the equally stringent ethical duties inscribed in moral codes are grounded in this clinical relationship. Informed consent is the first step in the groundwork for care, and it is more than a simple procedural act under a set of guidelines. Rather, consent is a sign of the implicit understanding between the physician and patient and the acceptance by both of the dyadic relationship to be crafted jointly. As is the case for any relationship, the backbone of the doctor-patient partnership is communication; yet in the clinical setting, this is not simply a form of reciprocal dialogue between equals. The physician has the overweening responsibility of attentive listening that is relational. In addition to the instrumental demands for information and direction necessary to medical care, this particular form of listening on the part of the physician is the means and the grounding for attending to the needs of the patient.

What makes the relational form of clinical listening different from informational and transactional listening and crucial to medicine? To start with, relational listening represents a receptive attentiveness to language and words that transmit meaning. The attention focused on the patient signals receptivity and creates a space in which the ill person's concerns can be expansively aired, thoughtfully considered, and gently interrogated. Attentive listening engages the full perceptual and cognitive capacity of the listener and involves the speaker, the utterance, and the listener. It demands knowledge of how language works and sensitivity to word choice, paralanguage, and the prosodic nuances of flow, pitch, hesitations, and pauses that may point to anxieties or to hidden concerns too difficult to articulate. The patient's narrative provides that individual's understanding of the genesis of the illness—the idiosyncratic logic of causality. The choice of "the" disease rather than "my" disease—serves to distance a feared diagnosis from the storyteller. And not to be neglected are the nonverbal cues and body language. Relational listening is reminiscent of hermeneutic readings of texts, with attention to subtexts, cryptic meanings, intricate allusions, as well as that which remains unsaid. This mode demands an open-mindedness to novelty and nuance, a keen awareness of inference, and comfort with eloquent silences. It also relies on a particular withholding of judgment, whether critique or affirmation, and a presumption that the other may be right. Tolerance and patience encourage an uninterrupted narration by the patient that is personal and idiosyncratic and offers an explanation for the genesis and course of the particular illness. Listening for information generally privileges ordinary daily language, whereas relational listening is attuned to figurative language and metaphoric framings. It seeks meaning in addition to information and permits exploration of issues across broader horizons. Attentive or relational listening may require the formation of new habits by the physician and an awareness of the variety of ways of seeing the world.

While attentive listening is akin to textual deciphering, the patient is not simply a document or text or image that challenges comprehension. The relational element posits necessarily that the patient is not an object but an individual who is an interlocutor and partner in the clinical dialogue. Thus, we must explore the affective, emotional, and ethical dimensions of relational listening that transcend the acquisition of simple, though crucial, diagnostic and demographic information. The interpersonal and social connections mediated by and dependent on language and listening distinguish the relational from the informational and make possible the enactment of compassionate clinical care. The stance of patience, focused and undivided attention, and acceptance of the value and validity of the story of the patient flattens the hierarchy and elides the paternalism that has historically tinged doctors' attitudes. It demonstrates that the concerns of the patient are being taken seriously and concurrently signals respect for the person who is speaking. Listening to a speaker entails recognition of that person; it generates the trust that is required for an unveiling of complex, difficult, and perhaps shameful or fearful beliefs. The dyadic partnership thus created is the forum for a co-construction of the narrative of illness as experienced by the patient and received and understood by the clinician.

One might reasonably consider the term "inattentive listening" as an oxymoron. Yet, patients commonly report unengaged, uninterested physicians who are turned away from them toward the computer screens, and too many tell of clinic visits in which they feel neglected, neither greeted nor examined and hardly offered eye-to-eye contact. In ordinary social interactions such behavior would be considered unseemly and rude, yet is apparently tolerated in today's harried hospitals and clinics. Inappropriate forms of clinical listening, let alone virtual neglect, are counterproductive in accomplishing the goals of the clinician (and patient) and, to add insult to injury, bespeak an arrogance and judgmentalism that undermine and abrogate the nascent dyadic partnership necessary to proper care.

Listening is not a passive act. It requires engagement and the exercise of specific skills and the clinical listener is no more a simple recipient than the textual critic is a simple reader. The philosopher Gemma Fiumara[6] has argued that persons do not listen when others speak—rather, speakers speak when listeners are present. She follows Socrates in using the term "maieutic," derived from a Greek word referring to obstetrics and midwifery, to describe the work of a listener who is giving birth to the nascent thoughts and words of the speaker. The listener is therefore an active participant in a genuinely creative and interactive engagement and assists in determining what the speaker will say. The bi-personal space made possible by the listener requires that individual's forbearance from speaking and permits the speaker to respond to the implicit invitation. Wittgenstein describes this space as "the 'temple' of a listening silence—which provides a background and does not interrupt."[7] This act of making room for the thoughts and words of the speaker demands a quality of attentiveness by the listener that Heidegger characterizes as "imperturbability,"[8] reminiscent of Sir William Osler's invocation of "aequanimitas." Fiumara reminds us of the bilaterality of the engagement and its relational character: "The message from the other will not attain its expressive potential except in the context of a relationship through which the listening interlocutor actually becomes a participant in the nascent thought of the person who is talking."[9] This entry into the psychic home of the other must be enacted with care and humility in order to avoid imposition and violence. Our Western tradition celebrates a form of communication that is expressive and emphatic, rather than one that is engaging and empathic.

The bilateral or relational nature of listening and speaking fostered by the maieutic act permits a genuine and honest sharing of thoughts and ideas that in turn enables the ethical dimensions of the clinician's role. Writing about his own experiences as a patient with a serious illness, the sociologist Arthur Frank speaks of "the story that I could not tell unless they listened,"[10] reflecting the maieutic role of the listener. He then describes the impact of this act, as follows: "When I as an ill person offer someone my story, I reach out as one human to another ... telling the story also implies a relationship that I desire with those who care for me."[11] Frank underlines that "embracing" the reciprocity is "the beginning of clinical work."[12] And why is that the case? Because to listen to stories is "to honor them" such that "the person who is so attended is no longer alone."[13] The choice of the word "attended" reflects the embedded meanings of listening, paying attention, and providing care, all framed by the obligations and duties of the clinician to the person who seeks help.

The reciprocal engagement may help us understand Aristotle's observation that hearing takes precedence over vision for "developing thought," echoed by the clinical teacher Howard Spiro: "The eye is for accuracy, but the ear is for truth."[14] Vision collects clinical information without the need for responsiveness by the person or object being examined. By contrast, attentive listening to a patient is an act of reciprocity and mutual recognition. The playwright and actor Anna Deavere Smith expressed this enactment in daily living, using a common understanding of the concept of empathy: "People speak of putting themselves into other people's shoes. My way of doing that is to put myself into other people's words. It all starts with listening."[15] To this keen observer of the human condition, entry into peoples' lives begins with listening to them and engaging with their words.

A study of healing relationships in primary care led by John Scott underscores the need for the physician's presence and the patient's desire to be known. A family physician extends the duties of the clinician to adapt the mode of engagement so as to respond to the specific needs of the patient, through the following reflections: "Is this a story of shame and they need you to listen? Is this a story of fear and they need you to be there with them? Is this a story of blame ... or self-blame and they need to hear that it wasn't their fault? I mean, what is the story? So what role do they need you to be in?"[16] The required sensitivity of a responsive clinical presence is grounded in a finely tuned and fully engaged capacity of deep listening. Keen and reflective attention provides the physician with the genre of the story that is being shared and the specific needs of the narrating patient at that given moment in time. The maieutic listener learns that some births are more difficult than others and may be aided by an adapted bedside presence.

A particular challenge for the clinical listener is to attend to the stories of patients who are reluctant to speak. In some instances, a sense of trust must be developed before difficult or intimate details can be readily shared. In others, a past experience of not having been heard or simply ignored has proven offensive or demeaning to a patient, who then shuts down and offers only superficial or trivial information in a later clinical encounter. The imperative for the physician in such circumstances is to hold back from an understandable inclination to fill the open conversational space and thereby prevent any effective engagement. Rather, the reflective listener will try to discern why the patient is reluctant to speak and will refrain from abrupt or intrusive demands. Psychiatrists have learned through their particular training and experience that silence on the part of the astute and attentive caregiver can be clinically effective in liberating the speech of the reluctant patient.

Goal Confusion and Role Confusion

If patients remind us of the imperative to be listened to and heard, and august professors of medicine from William Osler to present-day convocation speakers enjoin medical students to listen to their patients—why then are physicians routinely and perhaps even increasingly afflicted with clinical deafness? Physicians are well intentioned and dedicated to their patients, and the causes are thus likely to be structural rather than due to lapses in individual behaviors.

Two underlying mechanisms help clarify this paradox. One is goal confusion—that is, physicians and patients are working together but their attention and goals are directed to different outcomes and are not completely congruent. The doctor's training and inculcated motivations are to understand diseases in order to detect them through the process of diagnosis. This is the well-known and celebrated Sherlock Holmes construct of medicine—the famous fictional detective, modeled on an actual professor of medicine, aims to solve the crime and apprehend the criminal. While the aggrieved victim may thereby benefit, that is not a major concern for our Holmesian hero. The detective searches for method, motive, and opportunity, and his counterpart, the doctor, seeks to unearth the pathological mechanism, causal organism, and genetic susceptibility. The ill person, by contrast, seeks reassurance, recognition, and attention and desires to be healed and once again be made whole. The patient needs to know that the physician has listened, is personally engaged, and appreciates what is at stake for the individual seeking care. The sets of goals are not in opposition but focus attention on different objectives or end points and perhaps reflect different job descriptions. Goal confusion has been more formally described as disparate attentional anchors. This divergence of interests is illustrated in the comment from an articulate family physician: "In the process of differential diagnosis there is a well-tried clinical method for understanding diseases, but no equivalent method for understanding patients."[17]

The second source of incongruence between physicians and patients is role confusion or rhetorical divergence. The Western cultural model of a professional is a rational, clear-minded, and articulate person (generally, male) who can provide with confidence answers that are driven by data. These are the heroic physicians and victorious barristers of television dramas who can fill any silence and win any war. A contemporary figure is the now ubiquitous management consultant who can answer all questions for all seasons and for whom silence is tantamount to unemployment. For these professionals, the ability to speak is an imprimatur of status and renown and, at times, synonymous with performance and skill. An assured and declarative rhetorical style is so firmly embedded in the role description that a physician who does not speak is a contradiction in terms. In other words, a non-speaking doctor is a nonexistent figure—a ghostly palimpsest of the contemplative, concerned physician sitting by a patient's bedside depicted in Sir Luke Fildes' famous painting.

The patient, by contrast, yearns to be heard and acknowledged, whose fears must be assuaged. A story that is received as a gift honors the narrator who is thereby known and signals a listener worthy of trust. This relational bond permits the disclosure of vulnerabilities and enables recognition of the patient as a particular person rather than as a generic agglomeration of symptoms emblematic of a given disease. The narrative is more than the sum of laboratory information and imaging data. It is the story of a life interrupted and a narrator in distress—a tale that cannot be transmitted in a vacuum. The maieutic listener is midwife to the birth of the story and the enactment gives life to the patient.

These currently prevalent rhetorical tropes present us with an existential dilemma: a physician who does not speak does not exist, and a patient to whom one does not listen cannot exist. An authentic clinical medicine is constituted by a listening physician and a speaking patient—currently an existential impossibility. Little wonder that patients are unhappy and physicians burn out. The dearth of opportunities for affective and effective engagement and recognition is not due to ill-intentioned doctors but the incongruity of their culturally and linguistically constrained goals, roles, and monologic modes.

A False Dichotomy

The two rhetorical modes that contribute to the barriers that separate physicians and patients and impair effective and necessary dialogic understandings and mutual appreciation are themselves grounded in long-standing differences between the world views of the natural sciences and the humanities, the two inspirational wellsprings of medicine (please see Table 9.1: Two Ways of Knowing the World). This broad distinction permits us to analyze and distinguish between the two major frameworks of knowing the world that generally characterize the scholarly disciplines. The table compares the nature of scholarship and understanding of the natural sciences in the column on the left with the *Weltanschauung* of the humanities on the right. Medicine has most often been categorized with the natural sciences, and certainly the knowledge of diseases which forms the basis of modern medicine is firmly grounded in the natural and life sciences. Physicians are trained to regard themselves as bedside scientists whose goal is to search for diagnostic truth using the thought processes of logical deduction to ascertain the nature of the disease afflicting the patient. The data collected by observation, laboratory testing, and imaging are evaluated by the norms of the population and inductive statistical analysis. Thereafter, therapeutic interventions are selected in accordance with the rubrics of evidence-based medicine that is grounded in generalizable knowledge and compiles the outcomes of the best available clinical trials for a given condition. The scientific physician takes a stance with regard to the disease with the rhetorical aims of comprehension, detection, and elimination. The attitude is direct—it is cloaked in power and rooted in vision.

The patient lives in the world of illness and has a rather different array of descriptors to characterize the relevant experiences and needs. The person seeks help in discerning the meaning of the illness to the rudely interrupted life and its future. The

Table 9.1 Two Ways of Knowing the World

Natural Sciences	Humanities
Scientific	Hermeneutic
Physicians	Patients
Truth	Meaning
Generalizable	Idiographic
Direct	Relational
Diagnosis	Understanding
Therapy	Healing
Evidence-Based Medicine (EBM)	Narrative
Population	Individual
Power	Strength
Vision	Hearing

narrative of illness demands the method of the hermeneutic scholar in deciphering complex texts, and the mode of logic is that of abduction that aims to answer the idiographic question, "What antecedents and contextual conditions explain the situation in which we find ourselves now?" It is indeed the case that the power of science helps the physician understand the genetic mutation that may make certain persons susceptible to a certain environment or organism. But, the objective of the hermeneutic clinician is not to describe diseases but to understand the unique story of illness of the particular patient who seeks help in the moment. Or, to return to a clinician's formulation of the puzzle, "Why is this individual, with a specific genetic endowment, developmental history, and unique amalgam of life experiences, in my clinic today?" The answers must be idiographic, that is, relevant to the specific person who is the patient and can help the physician gain insights into the nature and course of illness and also respond to the multitude of questions that arise in the mind of the ailing individual. "Why am I sick? Will I get better? Why did this happen to me? Am I to blame? Did I do anything wrong? I am afraid of what may happen—is that normal?" The patient, as we have learned, seeks information, reassurance, and recognition. The person needs to be understood not as a case or instance of a model gleaned from a textbook, but as sui generis, unique unto the self. Understanding is more expansive than and encompasses diagnosis, and healing enriches therapeutic interventions. The desirable stance of the physician is relational rather than direct and strength replaces power. That is, the strength of the doctor is to withhold judgment and listen to the words and thoughts of the dyadic counterpart and the resilience of the patient is nurtured by the silence of the physician. Lastly, the most relevant sensory modality is hearing and its capacity of reciprocated understandings.

The apparent dichotomy between these two canonical ways of knowing the world has long been a feature of the discourse about and within medicine. It is recognizable in the debates on whether the Aristotelian virtues of techne or *phronesis* are more apt in characterizing medicine. In more prosaic terms, we hear discussions about medicine as a science or an art, about the doctor's head or heart as more germane to practice, and contemporary questions regarding the role of the humanities in the medical curriculum. Such disputes illustrate and aggravate the problem of what has been termed the "dual discourse of clinical medicine." The purported split between the natural sciences and the humanities are in actuality complementary modes of understanding the world and, rather than being oppositional, provide stereoscopic depth of comprehension. The false adversarial framing is one of a large array of dichotomies that afflict many disciplines and undermine coherent descriptions. Well-known examples in medicine include nature versus nurture, soma versus psyche, biomedical versus biopsychosocial, science versus art, physical versus psychosomatic, and competence versus compassion. The distinctions between these viewpoints are useful and appropriate for analysis and in order to decipher the origins of the sometime stark differences between the goals and roles of physicians and patients. At the same time, the fatal flaw of such dichotomization lies in the promulgation of a clinical medicine that cannot exist. That is, medicine without scientific grounding and generalizable knowledge cannot accomplish its goals of helping those who need care. Yet, the truths of science and the benefits of contemporary technology and pharmacology are bereft of their value if they are not brought to the bedside by a caring physician to a trusting patient within the humanized space of the clinical relationship. An interesting articulation of the complementarity of these two domains, that of the sciences and that of the humanities, was provided by the philosopher Giambattista Vico. He noted that when "sentences formed by reflection and reasoning rise towards universals, the closer they approach the truth." Whereas, the more "sentences formed by feelings of passion and emotion ... descend to particulars, the more certain they become."[18] In medicine, the entwinement of universals parsed out to the particularities of the individual patient constitute the basis for the clinical craft.

Speaking and Listening: Origins of an Imbalance

In her exploration of the philosophy of listening, Gemma Fiumara examines the Greek sources of our Western intellectual and cultural traditions. She compares the Greek words *logos*, referring to speech or expression, a particular utterance or assertion, and *legein*, which refers to speak or say and is also used in the sense of gather, receive, and bring together. While there is a large array of meanings for *logos* in addition to speech, there is a marked absence of references to a capacity for listening. Fiumara cites Martin Heidegger to make the point that the expressive aspect of *legein* has become predominant in the tradition we have inherited, and that the dialogic mode of *legein* has been suppressed by the monologic form of *logos* in our human interactions. She notes that our "power of expression ... is largely programmed for not listening"[19] and as a result we have become "masters of discourse" rather than "apprentices of listening."[20] We harbor the illusion that it is possible to speak with others without listening to them and we live with the misconception that we can form relationships in a monologic mode. In fact, we are now acculturated to competing monologues as surrogates for reciprocity. In consequence, Fiumara concludes, we gravitate toward metaphors of hunting and battle, and communication becomes a function of speech and expression shorn of a need for listening.

The absence of a capacity for listening is more than a simple loss of one of the two dimensions necessary to an interaction. It renders impossible the creation of the relationship that undergirds all human dyads, including the clinical interaction germane to the goals of medicine. Listening permits us to auscultate the thoughts of the other and not simply to capture a photograph of the body, reminiscent of the comparative values of hearing and vision. Gadamer sums it up eloquently: "Anyone who listens is fundamentally open. Without this kind of openness to one another there is no genuine human relationship. Belonging together always means being able to listen to one another."[21] Listening possesses a "binding function"[22] that demands strength, devotion, and perseverance, all rooted in humility.

Listening in Our Time

It is not difficult to enhance medical curricula with teaching sessions designed to develop communications skills and to provide simulation center training sessions on attentive listening. Such modules are now common in medical schools and are routinely required by guidelines and criteria for accreditation. While such interventions are recent, recognition of the importance of listening is evident in medical writings for over a century and articles on methods of teaching communication skills were readily available in the 1970s. Despite such widespread and diligent efforts, patients, students-in-training, and social critics continue to observe and report frequent lapses in appropriate attention and listening, while commenting on the importance of this clinical skill.

There are, most assuredly, structural barriers that stand in the way of achieving the attitudes and skills necessary to an effective clinical attentiveness responsive to the needs of our patients. Medicine is situated in noisy and cacophonous physical and social environments that are not conducive to a quiet exchange of information and concerns. It is not simply a matter of physical noise but also the overwhelming bombardment of auditory spam, much of it irrelevant yet disconcerting. We also witness a continuing loss of trust in science and intellectual expertise more generally—note the burgeoning cadres of opponents to vaccination and to public health measures more generally. This societal mistrust is mirrored by an equally pernicious tendency within medicine, namely the denigration of idiographic sources of understanding and an overweening emphasis on objectivity. The structures of hierarchy and power within medicine aggravate the social distance between patients and professionals, making it increasingly difficult to support an ethos of mutuality and transcend the necessary differences in expertise and needs with an egalitarian humility and humanity that foster compassion. Finally, achieving the requisite capacity for listening entails clearing a space in a Western culture with a millennial tradition that is deaf to this critical capacity for authentic engagement. Nurturing a capacity for listening demands personal psychological growth and adaptation and, more broadly, cultural realignment and evolution—simply adding curricular training will not be sufficient to the task at hand. And yet, the imperative is clear: listening is the armature of the clinical method that in turn is the conduit to fulfilling the mandates of healing and care.

10
A Pharmacology of Words

[A]n important lesson in physic is here to be learnt, the wonderful and pow-
erful influence of the passions of the mind upon the state and disorder of
the body. This is too often overlooked in the cure of disease.... what won-
derful effects the passions of hope and faith, excited by mere imagination,
can produce on disease.

—**John Haygarth,** *Of the Imagination as a Cause and*
as a Cure of Disorders of the Body, **1800**

The eminent physician of the British Enlightenment and Fellow of the Royal Society, John Haygarth, carried out what may have been the earliest investigation using a placebo and demonstrated that "false" wooden probes were as effective in the relief of symptoms as the highly popular metal models with their touted "galvanic properties." He was a careful observer and concluded, "What powerful influence upon diseases is produced by mere imagination."[1] Haygarth's careful analysis was an exception to the common wisdom at the beginning of the nineteenth century that a placebo was an emblem of deceit, and although the phrase "decipimur specie" (deceptive form) appears in a small font on his title page, he certainly understood the lesson for clinical medicine. Haygarth's contemporaries were rather more cynical, as exemplified in Quincy's *Lexicon-Medicum* of 1811, defining placebo as "a common place method" that "works not by assisting but by pleasing" the patient,[2] and in America, by Thomas Jefferson's allusion to pious fraud.[3] In non-medical sources, we find Placebo as the name of one of Chaucer's pilgrims, depicted as a flatterer and sycophant, contributing to the long-held and rather resistant concept that placebo, that is, pleasing the patient, was somehow wrong, if not shameful. Despite these denigrating assessments that placebos could do no more than please those who are ill without actual salutary benefits, they were used widely and routinely during the nineteenth and twentieth centuries. Indeed, recent surveys have shown that more than half of American internists and rheumatologists routinely use placebo treatments, though they do not necessarily divulge that to the patients offered such prescriptions.

The widespread use of placebo treatments in medicine notwithstanding, a lingering sense of deception and lack of transparency continue to undermine the understanding and application of this very powerful therapeutic modality. Hippocrates understood that "health may be implanted in the sick by certain gestures" and noted that both healing and disease "may be communicated from one to another,"[4] by human contact. Yet, two millennia later, the definition in the OED refers to placebo as an intervention "prescribed more for psychological benefit to the patient being given treatment than for any direct physiological effect ... [with] no specific therapeutic effect on a patient's condition."[5]

What explains the widespread use of placebos despite the skepticism and mistrust of such apparently innocuous interventions, even when placebos are shown to have potent benefits in clinical medicine? The belief among clinicians who prescribe placebos that patients must be unaware of these "fake" medicines in order to reap their benefits generates an aura of subterfuge that causes unease for some. Prescribing a placebo pill increases the physician's awareness of the ritual of practice and may spur a reminder, perhaps unwelcome to some clinicians, of the shamanistic roots of medicine. A sense of deceit may also hark back to the era of patent medicines and fraudulent marketing that began in eighteenth-century England and reached its peak in the snake-oil salesmen of the American Wild West in the late nineteenth century. These widespread, risky, and deceptive activities by charlatans spurred the establishment of the Food and Drug Administration in the United States, yet such practices never disappeared completely. Some of the hallmarks of the sideshow atmosphere resurfaced in the online hawking of panaceas during the COVID-19 pandemic.

A desire to leave behind this sordid history of false cures and illicit compounds was strengthened by the advent of scientific understanding of health and disease that became a burgeoning force in the field of medicine in the middle of the twentieth century. The growth of pharmacology and its array of powerful medicines and technical innovations led to dramatic reforms of health care and improved outcomes. In turn, societal trust in and reliance on medical care grew and strengthened over the past century of increasing life expectancy and effective modalities of care. Whether these benefits accrued from systems of public health, better sanitation, vaccination, and nutrition or from drugs and physicians—in any case, the public imagination has been thoroughly captivated by scientific achievements.

At the same time, the influence of science in medicine and medical education has had an unintended and unfortunate consequence of an increasingly reductionist understanding of the care of patients. A holistic view of persons, the contexts in which they live and the illnesses from which they suffer, has given way to a focus on the particular detail with its microcosmic views of causality and pathogenesis. As a result, physicians and those whom they teach have become increasingly inured to short visits, truncated narratives, and single-minded demands to order an invasive diagnostic procedure and prescribe a very specific medication, perhaps tailored to the patient's genetic markers. These shifts of emphasis, accelerated by the profit-driven motives of efficiency of the health care industry, have narrowed the medical gaze such that it can no longer encompass an embodied person with experiences in the context of family and community and the systems of beliefs accrued through life and living. This directed attention to subunits and away from broader frameworks of understanding suggests that the lenses of values, meanings, and cultures and the societal embeddedness of persons are no longer readily available. Without such expansive framings, placebos and their magical benefits lie beyond rational comprehension and become objects of suspicion and derision.

The instrumental use of inert placebos in clinical research as comparators to presumptively active novel drugs was an important methodological development that was foreshadowed by the experiments of the prescient Dr. Haygarth and became a routine element of drug trials in the second half of the twentieth century. This mode of comparison was revolutionary in the field of medical innovation in affording a measure of the specific effects of a new drug or surgical intervention, distinguished from the influences of the myriad incidental and nonspecific effects on subjects of the contextualized clinical trial process itself. The introduction of randomized, double-blind clinical trials contributed to the impressive pharmacological innovations in oncology and cardiology since 1950. This research process, however, brought with it unanticipated misconceptions that hampered an understanding of the therapeutic potential of placebos. Given that the results of placebo control arms of clinical trials are intended to be subtracted from the overall outcomes to showcase the actual benefits of the therapy being tested, placebos became regarded by some pharmacologists and trial designers as noise in the data or a nuisance that contaminates or masks the important findings. More to the point is the inevitable disdain for placebos as inert substances whose only purpose is to eliminate false conclusions about drug efficacy and highlight the value of pharmaceutical creativity. The understanding of placebos as inert substances without physiological effects that are stand-ins for background noise in blinded trials promoted a skepticism that added to concerns about deception. In other words, the entirely appropriate practice of informing subjects and gaining their consent to the use of placebos as controls in clinical trials inevitably highlighted the ethical concerns about the absence of consent to such interventions in daily clinical practice. As a consequence, while placebos in clinical research were understood as inert but necessary and acceptable, their use in practice was viewed with suspicion and some disdain, as in the phrases, "it's only a placebo" and "it can neither hurt nor help." The property of inertness (it cannot help) tainted the stance necessary for benefit in daily clinical work (it may help). A more egregious result of such language is the apprehension of some patients that any benefits from placebos, whether in trials or medical care, would lead their physicians to conclude that "it's all in your head," that is, neither the illness nor the unexpected benefits of the inert placebo are real, only imagined. Apart from creating misunderstandings about placebos and their utility, this attitude toward placebos fosters confusion, and perhaps anger, for many patients who conclude that their doctors care little about them and the symptoms that concern them. Placebos as control elements and comparators in clinical trials generate the expectation that any beneficial or salutary responses cannot be real or meaningful, since their very value to the trial designer is their very inertness, or, in the instance of sham surgery, the word itself suggests their non-validity. Thus, consent forms that necessarily describe placebos as inert and surgery as sham inadvertently denigrate the very nature of placebos. The widespread, though erroneous, understanding that placebos are pills, that is, necessarily physical substances, undermines the idea that what counts is not a placebo as object but rather as process and, perhaps, as ritual.

Thus, three significant developments of the second half of the twentieth century, each an important contributor to contemporary medicine—namely, biomedical scientific research, randomized clinical trials, and informed consent—contributed, unintentionally and perhaps paradoxically, to widespread skepticism regarding placebos and to their shady reputation in the public imagination.

Medical students invariably ask whether the use of placebos entails lying to patients. They are genuinely concerned about the ethical dimensions of treatments and prescriptions and effectively mirror current cultural perspectives. This viewpoint generates at least two questions for consideration: How can we account for the skepticism common among medical students and their later routine use of placebos in clinical care? Second, how are these various paradoxes regarding placebos relevant to the language of medicine and the care of patients?

What Are Placebos?

Placebo treatments in clinical research are interventions with no known pharmacological activity, that is, inert substances or actions intended to serve as control conditions in evaluating the efficacy of novel drugs or procedures. Their impact (placebo response) can be assessed in a study by comparing the status of subjects or patients before and after the placebo intervention. Alternatively, in some trial designs, the placebo effect is measured by comparing subjects or patients enrolled in a placebo group with those in a no-intervention arm. Some researchers in the field of placebos make a useful distinction between the two modes of comparison just noted. Before-and-after differences could be the result of the specific placebo pill or intervention but may also reflect other ongoing background or contextual circumstances. For example, the illness in question could wax or wane, repeated statistical measurements can fluctuate, outliers may regress to the mean, and the interactions of subjects with persons or the environments in which the investigations are being conducted could lead to changes during the course of the trial. Thus, the placebo *response* noted in pre- and post-comparisons is a combination of the specific effects of the placebo and all the other contextual impinging factors. When a placebo arm is compared to a no-intervention arm, all the contextual effects should be the same in both arms, and the differences in outcomes are attributed to the placebo per se and labeled the placebo *effect*. In clinical practice, placebo responses are changes in symptoms and signs following placebo treatments that cannot be attributed to any known pharmacological properties of the agent or intervention. Once again, such responses are the result of the combination of the impact of the pill or intervention and all the ancillary factors that contribute to the evolution of illness and the results of all clinical interactions. The importance of these distinctions will become clearer when we return to the importance of context and persons in clinical therapeutics.

The interest in placebos in medicine beyond their use as controls in clinical research stems from recurrent observations in many settings and in trials of a variety of interventions that beneficial responses are evident in about 30% of subjects enrolled in the placebo arms of clinical trials for a diverse array of clinical conditions. In the subjects who demonstrate a placebo response, the improvement may be as much as 50% of that elicited by the active pain medication, for example. Such significant findings are most common in trials for treatment of acute and chronic pain, depression, low back pain, and fatigue, including in persons with cancer. More surprising, perhaps, were similar observations of reduction of pain and discomfort in patients in the control arms of surgical interventions for cardiac angina, osteoarthritis of the knee, back pain, and gastric reflux. In many instances, especially in research on depression and pain, the overall differences between the active-intervention arm and the placebo arm are of minor clinical importance and most of the beneficial outcomes are attributable to the placebo response rather than the active agent being investigated. Of greater interest is the steadily growing proportion of subjects with beneficial responses to placebos in trials for management of pain or depression carried out during the past three decades. In other words, placebos seem to be getting better! The impressive and clinically significant responses to placebos used for many common conditions associated with debilitating pain and suffering for so many patients finally led to a turn in thinking among clinicians and researchers from a focus on placebos as elements of control conditions for trials to a serious consideration of placebos of various kinds as potential therapeutic agents. The aim of these clinical investigators is not simply to demonstrate what was already known, that placebos provide benefits to many patients, but rather to parse the placebo responses to understand how such improvements come about and what beyond the inert drug or intervention is responsible for these effects.

Not surprisingly, many investigators quickly showed that the evident benefits were not due to the inert substance but rather the surroundings and contextual circumstances: the person administering or providing the medication, the practices and rituals associated with the intervention, and the attitudes of both the persons receiving and providing care. Thirty years ago, a British family physician reported that two thirds of his patients seeking help for minor yet troubling symptoms improved after he provided reassurance and what he termed a "positive consultation." By contrast, only a third of a similar group of patients who received a neutral, noncommittal consultation experienced a lessening of symptoms. At the same time, a prescription of a placebo vitamin pill had no useful effect compared with those leaving without a prescription. His conclusion: the placebo benefit is derived not from the pill but the supportive and positive attitude of the physician.[6]

A similar outcome resulted from a more elaborate trial examining three components of the placebo response in patients with irritable bowel syndrome.[7] One group of patients was enrolled on a waiting list and did not receive any specific trial interventions. A second group received a series of sham acupuncture treatments and the third cohort received the same series of sham acupuncture interventions (needles that do not penetrate the skin) and, in addition, an extended 45-minute friendly and supportive consultation with the acupuncturist. Symptoms were then carefully assessed over a span of several weeks, and all three groups improved. Even the group on the waiting list got better, presumably because of the interactions with investigators during enrollment and perhaps an expectation of benefit. However, the most impressive and most durable lessening of symptoms and improvements of quality of life were evident in the patients who were the beneficiaries of a supportive and sympathetic clinical interaction. Indeed, in some instances the improvements lasted for six weeks, and extended beyond the period of active interventions. Thus, all the putative elements of a placebo response were helpful to the patients—the anticipation of treatments, a sham intervention, and a caring practitioner. Once again, the third of these elements, the human administering care appears to provide the most potent and longest-lasting contribution to relief of symptoms and patient satisfaction.

A finely grained dissection of components of placebo responses was conducted with normal subjects using allergic skin reactions induced by local administration of small doses of histamine.[8] These routinely cause skin reactions (wheals) whose magnitude can be readily measured. The application of a placebo cream to the injection site reduced the size of the wheal in those subjects who were told to expect improvements from the cream but not in those who were warned to expect worsening. Furthermore, improvements following the presentation of positive expectations were significantly enhanced by signs of warmth and competence on the part of the participating health care providers. By contrast, subjects faced with negative expectations showed no such beneficial responses to warmth and competence. The beneficial placebo response elicited by verbal expectations is most effectively generated and strengthened by caregivers whose behaviors display warmth and competence. Thus, clinical good is more readily evoked and enhanced by human interactions with caregivers than by the inert medication or sham process alone.

The domain of complementary and alternative medicine produces results that support these ideas. In one study, patients with active, stable rheumatoid arthritis receiving conventional treatments were enrolled in a double-blind trial comparing the effects of homeopathic remedies with a personalized, detailed consultation with a practitioner of homeopathy.[9] While the homeopathic medicines were not helpful, the consultations led to significant clinical benefits including decreases in joint swelling, reduction of pain, and improved mood among the patients. The improvements following consultations were greater than those elicited by other nonpharmacological treatments for rheumatoid arthritis, including cognitive behavioral therapy. This study, from a very different realm of therapeutic practice, namely homeopathy, adds to the accumulating evidence in the field of placebos that the benefits accrue from an extended and supportive encounter with a caregiver and not from the chemically inert remedy.

The next shift in attention away from placebos as inert pills toward an analysis of the demonstrated clinical benefits came from innovative research designs that obviated the need for sugar or lactose pills and sham interventions.[10] The studies compared hidden administration of analgesics with open treatments that ordinarily constitute standard clinical care.[11] Patients requiring pain relief following surgical procedures were assigned to receive standard doses of pain medications via intravenous administration, but the individuals were not informed when the drug treatments were initiated as they were administered via a hidden pump. A second group of similar patients received the same drug treatments but were informed by a clinician in the room when the treatments were begun, as would be the case in routine care. In the setting of openly announced infusions, the onset of relief was almost immediate, and pain was measurably reduced within the first hour of infusion. In the covertly treated group, patients did not attain the same level of relief until three hours had elapsed. Conversely, when patients were informed that the analgesic infusion was stopped, pain increased after an hour, whereas pain relief continued for four hours when the termination of analgesia was covert. A lower dose of pain relief medication was required to cause a 50 percent reduction in pain for informed patients compared with hidden administration. This also reflects the finding in a traditional placebo comparison trial of pain relief for extraction of third molars in which a moderate dose of morphine was equivalent to a saline infusion administered by a clinician telling the patient that a potent analgesic is being injected.[12] Similar clinical responses to open but not covert administration of interventions were evident in management of postoperative anxiety and in open-versus-hidden modifications to deep brain stimulation in patients with Parkinson's disease and therapeutically implanted electrodes.[13]

This open/covert research paradigm is interesting for a number of reasons. It eliminates the need for a placebo pill or sham intervention and all patients or subjects receive active, standard treatments. There is no need to deceive the participants into thinking they will receive active treatments when that is not the case. The analytic value of the design is based on the following premise. Providing treatments can have two categories of benefits (or side effects): those due to the pharmacological properties of the drug or the physiological effects of a surgical intervention on one hand, and, on the other, a large assembly of influences that comprise, among others, knowledge and expectations on the part of the patient based on prior experience or those inculcated or elicited by the clinician, associative learning, conditioning, contextual properties of the treating environments, the comfort or security afforded by a clinical presence, and the patient's desire and hopes for improvement and healing. This second category of variables is sometimes referred to as *nonspecific*, though the term represents our lack of knowledge on the mechanisms of causality and not the lack of importance of such factors. Thus, open administration provides both categories of agency whereas covert or hidden provision of the same drugs eliminates all effects that fall into the second group of contributors. Of course, another term for this second grouping is the placebo! Therefore, this open/covert format provides a measurable assessment of the placebo response without the need for the inert agents themselves. A more significant element of this design is that it showcases all the attendant influences, what the influential physician Michael Balint has called the "atmosphere of the situation," that always accompany not only placebos but, significantly, the routine and daily use of any and all drugs and interventions of medical care. What we term *placebo responses* are an inevitable and important part of caregiving, including those clinical interactions that may not include pharmacological agents. The impressive results that emerge from the open/covert comparisons indicate the potency of all these nonspecific interactions and point to the need for a more careful dissection of what these are and how they achieve their benefits for patients, and their physicians.

If important clinical benefits are the result of influences that may be described as the placebo response, it behooves us to better understand the nature of such forces and processes and learn how they can be used to advantage. This entails deciphering how they accomplish their outcomes. Of course, we must also unearth the relationships among such contexts and processes and the words and language of the clinic.

But a first step is to describe research that helps us deal with the long-standing ethical conundrum of placebos as deceptive practice. Just as the open/covert paradigm permitted, paradoxically, the study of placebos without the need for inert pills or sham procedures, the interesting work on open-label placebos permits us to address the ethical dilemma.

The benefits evident in the use of placebos in a number of illnesses, the impressive effects of informing patients of the details of the treatments they are receiving in the open/covert designs, together with the ever-present concerns regarding truthtelling in clinical care, all combined to lead many investigators to examine the value of open-label placebos. In other words, a schema in which patients or subjects are told that they will receive a placebo treatment, generally described in positive terms, but not promising success. In some trials, the presentation is simply an envelope labeled "Placebo" and containing pills with instructions on administration. In trials of illnesses for which placebo arms have shown benefits, the open introduction might indicate that placebos have previously been helpful for patients with the same condition. In most instances, what seemed to be sufficient was a mildly optimistic and honest proposal that these placebo pills may help, so let's try them and see. Pointedly omitted were the previously common language of negativity and the stress on the inertness of placebos. Parenthetically, in light of the accumulating reports of the demonstrable benefits of placebo pills and interventions, one could make the case that emphasizing the impossibility of clinical improvements from placebos would constitute a deceptive statement! One of the earliest pilot studies of placebos, in 1965, was in the treatment of mild psychiatric illness—patients were told that sugar pills may help their condition. Indeed, fourteen of fifteen patients improved after a week of sugar pills taken three times a day.[14] The authors commented on the importance of non-blind research—yet, it took fifty years for the times to be deemed ripe for larger studies of open-label placebos. Over the span of a few years, studies appeared demonstrating the efficacy of such interventions in irritable bowel syndrome, depression, allergic rhinitis, acute migraine headaches, and chronic low back pain and in patients who had completed treatments for cancer yet had residual fatigue. In this last example, three weeks of placebo pills taken twice daily reduced fatigue and led to improved quality of life.[15] Thus, placebo responses do not require placebo pills, nor do they depend on subterfuge.

How Do Placebos Work?

The investigation of placebo actions by the methods of the neurosciences, including pharmacology and functional imaging of the brain, have helped decipher the seemingly mysterious effects of these long-practiced interventions. The research demonstrates that the body mechanisms known to play a role in the action of effective drugs are also active in the effects of placebos. In addition, the specific biological systems in play are those involved in the illness or biological phenomenon in question. For example, a locally applied placebo cream, described verbally to the subjects as a local anesthetic, provides relief from pain induced at a skin site by a small injection of an irritant. The relief is specific to the site at which placebo cream is applied, and pain at other skin sites with concurrent injections is not affected. When the opioid antagonist naloxone is administered intravenously, the effect of the placebo cream is blocked and no analgesic benefit is reported by the subjects. These findings suggest that the effect of the placebo cream is mediated by the body's endogenous opioid systems whose effects are blocked by naloxone. However, these endogenous opioids do not change the pain sensation at all injection sites but only at those treated with placebo cream. Thus, the effect of these endogenous natural analgesics is directed to, or elicited at, the local site at which the placebo cream is applied—this local effect is in turn generated by the subject's expectation of pain relief stimulated by the belief that an anesthetic cream has been administered. The expectation elicited by the verbal introduction and subsequent application of the placebo cream engages neurochemical mechanisms that are normally activated by analgesic drugs and presumably used in natural pain control systems. What the investigators refer to as "spatially directed expectancy,"[16] that is, the anticipation by the subjects that pain relief will be apparent specifically at the site of the placebo cream application, is itself the result of the language, both verbal and enacted, of the researchers in the experiment, together with prior lived experiences of the subjects. This conclusion adds to our accumulating evidence that placebos are a phenomenon of linguistically mediated or, more accurately, semiotically mediated human interactions.

Patients with Parkinson's disease may also respond well to a placebo, whether a pill or sham manipulation of electrodes implanted in the brain as part of a treatment regimen. In such trials, placebo interventions may improve motor function usually impaired in such persons. By contrast with pain studies, these improvements are due to the release of dopamine in the brain areas known to be damaged in Parkinson's disease.[17] The amount of dopamine released mirrors the extent of the placebo-induced improvement and is presumably due to the expectation of clinical improvement generated by the placebo. Thus, the physiological mechanisms by which placebos achieve their effects depend on the specific illness in question and how usual treatments for the malady accomplish their beneficial actions. For example, in Parkinson's disease, the therapeutic mainstays work by increasing the levels of dopamine in specific areas of the brains of patients—the same regions that exhibit the release of dopamine in response to placebos.

The same chemically innocent placebo, say, a sugar pill or saline infusion, can activate different neural mechanisms when used to represent different therapies or in different disease models or experiments. For example, prior conditioning can lead to an association between administration of morphine and a saline infusion. Subsequent pain relief by administration of saline can be inhibited by naloxone, indicating that the saline provided analgesia by evoking endogenous opioid release. An association between a non-opioid drug, ketorolac, that also possesses analgesic properties and a saline infusion can also be conditioned such that the saline administration relieves pain. In this instance, however, the benefit of the saline cannot be blocked by naloxone. Thus, the same placebo, saline, used to relieve pain in the same experimental model, utilizes different biological mechanisms to achieve the outcome, which depend on the specific circumstances of the prior conditioning. When the placebo response is elicited not by conditioning but the expectation motivated by an injection of saline announced as morphine, the resultant pain relief can be abrogated by naloxone. Even without prior conditioning, an expectation of analgesia elicits endogenous opioid mechanisms and an expectation of pain relief from saline previously conditioned to morphine enhances the analgesia that is completely blocked by naloxone. By contrast, a verbally triggered expectation of pain relief from saline that was conditioned to the non-opioid ketorolac also increases the analgesia that results from the ketorolac-conditioned saline alone, but, in that case, the effect is only *partly* reversed by naloxone. This work demonstrates a number of important features of placebos. Not surprisingly, the specificity of action and the actual biological mechanisms evoked cannot be the result of saline per se but are due to the biological responses elicited by the mode of induction. That is, when saline is associated with morphine by either expectation or conditioning, its effect is mediated by endogenous opioid systems. When saline is associated with ketorolac only by conditioning, opioid systems are not activated but currently unknown and apparently non-conscious mechanisms are responsible. However, when the ketorolac-conditioned saline is enhanced by cognitively transmitted expectations, part of the benefit, presumably that portion due to expectation of analgesia, is due to opioid systems and the balance due to these other, unknown neurochemical mediators.[18] Therefore, the same placebos work by different means depending on the illness in which they are used, for example, postoperative pain compared with Parkinson's disease, and the means by which the responses are evoked. While sugar pills and saline infusions are generic and hence nonspecific, what makes their actions very directed and specific are the mediators of the response—the interactions between physicians/investigators and patients/subjects and the triggering mechanisms thereby elicited. Perhaps more accurately in the clinical arena, the specificity derives from an interplay between the minds/bodies of the patients and those of the physicians and the various mediating elements thus engaged. The actual biological modes of action of placebos depend greatly on the context of presentation; the prior experience of the subjects or patients, whether by formal conditioning, lived events, or cultural assumptions; the intentions and behaviors of the persons providing the placebos; and the language, both verbal and semiotic, of the various human actors at play.

Modes of Elicitation

The behavioral or psychological means by which placebos engage the neurochemical and biological mechanisms that lead to the outcomes, whether experimental or clinical, in subjects or patients, respectively, require the communication or transmission of information. The actual pills or infusions do not alone specify the given outcomes or the mediating mechanisms—it thus follows that some information-laden signs must accompany or mediate in the placebo process. For example, in the open/covert comparison, the more effective analgesia of open administration appears to be due to the information provided to the patients regarding the administered infusions and perhaps also to the caregivers providing the placebo and the message. In the case of open-label placebos, the benefits may stem from the knowledge offered by the clinician or investigator that such pills have helped others and a transmitted feeling of confidence or optimism. In all instances, words, body language, signs, or other modes of information transfer are necessary to achieve the intended effects. The actual means by which signs and words affect the mind/body of a recipient are the focus of many streams of investigation and several models have been proposed to explain the behavioral and biological results. Perhaps the earliest to be developed empirically is the association of signals and physiological events by psychological conditioning made famous by Ivan Pavlov. Similar experiments exploring placebo effects have been carried out in animals in which drugs that dampen immunological responses in rats were linked by conditioning to flavored water that could then substitute for the drug in reducing immune responses in the conditioned animals. While similar phenomena have been noted in conditioning experiments with opioids and selected hormonal responses, formal conditioning is not thought to be a likely explanatory mechanism for most placebo effects, as these are readily evident in experimental and clinical settings in which there has been no prior conditioned linkage between the placebo and a biologically active agent. To cite only one example, sham knee surgery for osteoarthritis leads to improvements in patients with no previous history of any surgical operations.

However, other modes of experience can forge associations that may establish symbolic and linguistic linkages between previously unrelated elements. A useful descriptor for such experiential modalities is the term "associative learning."[19] Pavlovian conditioning is a formalized process of learning, but there are, in addition, more pragmatic and informal means of interacting with and fostering connections between persons and the world. Three modes of associative learning—personal, social, and cultural—warrant consideration.

Personal associative learning describes how we acquire knowledge of our world and, more particularly, how we connect events, features of our environment, and interactions with people and objects and then encode in memory these linkages of correlation and causality. Perhaps the best-known literary example is from Marcel Proust, who described the "involuntary memories" of his childhood experiences evoked by a simple madeleine, a French cake, that reflected an association formed many decades before its recall. This act of remembrance was infused with a powerfully affective sense of joy—an instance of a simple culinary placebo eliciting a strong biological response. In 1896, Dr. John McKenzie of Baltimore described the onset of "paroxysms" of sneezing and congestion induced by an artificial rose in a patient with seasonal allergies to hay and roses.[20] He referred to the "role of pure psychical impressions" in evoking clinical reactions. Practical, real-world clinical instances abound: an infant with experiences of illness, who begins to cry and fuss as soon as the technician in the hospital arrives to take yet another blood sample; a woman who becomes nauseous on entering the oncology day center for a scheduled infusion of chemotherapy; and a sufferer with a toothache who feels relief on arrival at the dentist's office and wonders why she insisted on an emergency appointment. These three examples share a feature not readily apparent in the Proustian instance, in that they demonstrate an expectation on presentation of the harbinger of an anticipated effect. All persons gather such associations in processes of learning that, by providing a portent of the immediate future, reduce uncertainty and permit rapid responses to instances of threats. Often, these learned reactions trigger autonomic fight-or-flight reactions, as in the child fearful of yet another needle-prick, or, a presumed evocation of endogenous opioid release by words or contextual signs when pain relief is gratefully anticipated. Other times, such communications of what is to come are unwelcome, for example, in studies that show that when a child or adult is warned that the forthcoming injection "won't hurt a bit," the actual discomfort and apprehension are heightened—an example of words as *nocebos*, the unhappy twin of placebos. In addition to foreshadowing what is to come, such learned signs and their associations permit a focus of attention and narrowing of perceptual purview to select those sensory inputs determined by experiences, whether personal or sociocultural, most relevant to a person's welfare and well-being. Even something as apparently straightforward as the perception of natural colors, for example, of fruits, is modulated by our prior experiences and the learned expectations of the colors we anticipate from an initial view of the shape of the object. An object in the shape of a banana appears more yellow than objects of unrelated contours.[21] Thus, our daily interactions with our environments (and one another) are the results of the specific sensations modulated by prior experiences and their associative learnings that shape our perceptions, cognitions, and embodied selves.

The social mode of associative learning is by observing others rather than by direct personal experience. An important example is the power of role models in education

and, in particular, the shaping effects of the hidden curriculum in medical education. Both admirable clinical teachers and, more rarely, those whose behaviors are less
than appropriate provide strong learning opportunities for impressionable and astute
medical students and residents-in-training. A second potent group of role models
are those encountered during childhood development: parents, siblings, playmates,
and teachers, among others, and, of course, such learning includes the acquisition of
language. Of clinical interest are the experiences of patients who observe others in a
shared hospital or health care environment responding well to interventions. Such
persons are more likely to associate and anticipate benefits from the same caregivers,
similar interventions, or simply from the treating environment itself. This phenomenon of social learning is confirmed by laboratory studies in which subjects demonstrated analgesic placebo responses to light stimuli whether they were formally
conditioned or simply acquired by witnessing other subjects showing such benefits.
The strengths of placebo analgesia were the same whether induced by conditioning
or social associative learning. Social learning may be operative in the effectiveness of
open-label placebos in those clinical settings in which they are seen to be helpful to
others and are also presented as beneficial by caregivers. By contrast, when placebos
are described to subjects in clinical trials, they are referred to as "neutral pills" that
should have no effect. The latter example can also constitute a socially learned nocebo.

Cultural learning involves neither personal experience nor direct observations.
Rather, the linkages are learned from a broader net of information sources. Some
associations are acquired formally through education, readings, and other conduits
of experiencing the world of ideas and people. It is likely that such culturally acquired
knowledge accounts for popular and experimentally verified notions that skin creams
have local effects, two placebo pills are better than one, pills taken three times a day
are more effective than single daily use, seemingly different placebos over the course
of several weeks are more effective than continuing the same formulation, big pills
are stronger, injections are more helpful than pills, and machine-dependent interventions and surgeons are the most potent agents in the hierarchy. The pharmaceutical
industry in the West has long known that sedatives work best when provided in pale
pastel colors, pink or blue, and uppers or stimulants should be red, orange or yellow.
Marketing on television and social media are significant rhetorical sources that shape
behaviors, including placebo responses. In trials of antihistamines, the subjects in the
placebo arm have stronger responses if they had been primed by television advertisements for treatments for seasonal allergies, even though they are not themselves
overtly aware of the effect.[22] Similarly, placebos provided in bottles labeled with well-
known brand names are more effective than generic labels, and as previously noted,
as the general public has become increasingly aware of antidepressant medications
through popular books and the press, the placebo responses in trials of antidepressants have increased steadily over several decades. Finally, comparisons of drug trials
conducted in different countries reveal impressive differences in placebo responses
that vary with the country and the specific illnesses being investigated, all attesting to
the contextual embeddedness of this important clinical phenomenon.

Rituals and Social Communication

The ritual of healing is practiced universally, yet its details and meanings are local and particular. Rituals may be formal and ceremonial or part of daily life and work, yet they are imbued with and dependent on words and signs, that is, modes of communication.

An enlightening description of the ritual of healing in the Native American Navajo nation by Ted Kaptchuk provides an important perspective on the power of symbolically laden human interactions. This pioneer in research on placebos in clinical care concludes that "placebo effects are the 'specific' effects of healing rituals."[23] Healing rituals are potent enactments whose power stems from theatrical dramas whose words and symbols enfold the patient or sufferer into a cultural allegory in which the healer's craft creates "an 'osmotic' bridge between cultural mythos and idiosyncratic biography."[24] The elements by which these ceremonies unfold in Navajo rituals are the same that support contemporary Western clinical engagements, namely, "metaphors and symbols, the healer's prestige, social interactions with relatives and community members ... performance of the ritual, and gesture, recitation, costume, iconography, touch, ingestion and the physical ordeal."[25] Moreover, these healing dramas depend on the active participation of the sufferer, who arrives with a desire to be treated and healed and who brings expectations, hopes, and desires that permit a transmogrification through ritual of the imagined into the real. The underlying mechanisms are the neurobiological and neurochemical networks of the brain evoked by words, symbols, and rituals. It will not surprise medical anthropologists, and ought not be a revelation to clinicians, that the cultural enactments of humans find their resonances in the activities of the embodied mind/brain and the lived reality of the person, in both sickness and health.

An epidemiological study of daily mortality rates from heart disease among Chinese and Japanese Americans living in California found a significant peak on the fourth day of the month, whereas no such increase was noted among a group of Caucasian matched controls.[26] In fact, for deaths attributed to chronic heart disease, the mortality rates among Chinese and Japanese Californians on the fourth day of the month were 27% higher than the monthly average. The belief that the number 4 is an unlucky omen and is avoided by many in China and Japan is attributed to a linguistic resemblance between the word for 4 that is a near homophone for the word for death in Mandarin, Cantonese, and Japanese. By contrast, the number 13, which is considered unlucky in some Caucasian societies, is not due to a linguistic resonance but has other cultural roots. The biological power of this cultural association is expressed and articulated in language and results in a potent nocebo phenomenon.

Several frameworks have been described to explain how learned associations, whether acquired by conditioning, personal, social, or cultural learning, influence minds/bodies through the mediation of words and language. These modes of learning are overlapping rather than completely distinct yet emphasize different aspects of the placebo/nocebo phenomenon. Individuals anticipate certain outcomes, pain relief, for example, when exposed to specific words or other contextual triggers previously linked to analgesia. Such expectations may be generated in the open arm of an open/ covert comparison by the words and body language of the investigator or the attitude and concerns of a clinician using an open-label placebo. This mechanism may indeed play a major role in laboratory research with healthy subjects, as we are all accustomed to situations in which we learn to expect discomfort, drowsiness, or arousal. The situation may differ somewhat and take on added complexity when working with persons who are actual patients with illness. Interviews with patients who have been subjects of placebo trials to alleviate symptoms of their illnesses do not describe a sense of expectation of improvement. Rather, they report a desire to get better, and a guarded optimism, that after many previous disappointments, this new approach, even one labeled "Placebo," may offer a benefit. In other words, not a rational expectation but an attitude of hope proffered by a therapeutic setting and a trusted physician. Some have referred to hope as an amalgam of a desire motivated by context, ritual, and belief allied with a more probabilistically rooted expectation generated by prior learning and experience. Stephen Jay Gould eloquently articulated this particular combination in his essay, "The Median Isn't the Message." He noted that the survival curve of mesothelioma, his own illness, had a long tail indicating a small but significant subgroup of patients with a rather long survival. This probability coupled to a clear desire to live and a Jamesian "Will to Believe" led to Gould's conviction that his own future would place him squarely in that long survival cohort.[27] He turned out to be appropriately optimistic in his hoped-for outcome when he lived two decades beyond the median eight-month survival for the rare tumor.

A different yet allied description focuses not on the psychological states of expectation or anticipation or hope but on the nature of the words, objects, and events that may elicit placebo (and nocebo) responses. This is the concept of meaning developed by Daniel Moerman[28] to capture those connotations of elements of the world that have particular resonances for one or more persons. Such elements have linguistic or semiotic, that is, symbolic content, and can elicit thoughts, memories, and affective states and thereby influence our minds/bodies. These words and symbols are the mediators between persons and the worlds in which they live, and such links between the social and the biological are reflected in the word "sociosomatics,"[29] coined by the medical anthropologist Arthur Kleinman to describe "the fundamental dialectic between the body and the social world."[30] We are aware of the influences of pills, infusions, colors, and sounds as symbolic elements embedded with meanings and the effect of the words of a ritual of healing or a voodoo ceremony with malign intent. Miller and Colloca have provided a list of examples of words and contexts relevant to the clinical setting that illustrate the concept of meaning, as follows: "clinician's white coat, diagnostic instruments, the appearance of the doctor's office or hospital room, the words communicated by the physician, the physician's disposition in listening and responding to the patient, gestures, and touch."[31] Such connotations may be idiosyncratic or shared only by certain patients, for example, the evocation of nausea by the chemotherapy infusion rooms, or the antipathy to tattoos by persons who experienced the markings of radiation therapy. Persons come to new experiences with the influences or baggage of prior life events. For families with memories of happy childbirths, driving by the hospital is a reminder of joy, while for others, clinical buildings are best avoided. Words and symbols differ in their connotations from one patient to another. Furthermore, different social and cultural roots inculcate meanings that may be cryptic to those of another ethnic or social group, and patients and physicians may not share or even be aware of one another's allusions and meanings. This is a reminder to clinicians of a need for tolerance, patience, and a will to listen and understand the elements of their patients' worlds and the resonances they evoke.

The receptivity of the mind/body to the connotations of symbols laden with prior experiences and memories help us understand the power of words and signs and the importance of the messengers and conduits of presentation. Placebos owe part of their power to actual bodily enactments and behaviors. It is not sufficient for patients to be offered placebos in open-label trials; to reap benefits they must actually take the pills even when they know them to be inert. An impressive demonstration of the importance of adherence in placebo responses is a meta-analysis by Scot Simpson and colleagues of a series of clinical trials examining the impact of adherence to drug regimens.[32] The overall risk of mortality among patients taking the study drugs as prescribed in these large trials was lower by half compared to those patients who did not follow the recommendations. That per se is not surprising. However, the same reduction of mortality risk by almost half was also noted in the subjects in control arms taking the placebos as prescribed compared to those who were non-adherent. Thus, engaging in one element of the enacted ritual of medicine, namely, taking the medication, is a requisite to gaining the benefit of the seemingly inert placebo pills or procedures.

The transmission of the words or symbols, that is, the meanings of the placebos, need not entail conscious awareness by the subject of the link between invocation and outcome. The associations that result from experiential learning do not necessarily depend on awareness and can be embodied and automatic. Conditioned associations can be learned subliminally and evoked by non-conscious triggers. These features indicate that when patients seek help and advice from their physicians, they arrive with a complex network of prior experiences and learned associations, some operating outside explicit conscious awareness, that endow the words, cues, and signals they encounter with particularized meanings and may evoke an embodied readiness for healing and relief. Similarly, previous unfortunate or unhappy experiences can precipitate a readiness for a complex encounter, fraught with misunderstandings, nocebo responses, and aggravation of the illness. The subliminal nature of such associations adds to the burden of the physician from whom help is sought, as important reactions of patients may not be readily understood without a careful, thoughtful, and delicately inquisitive stance by the caregiver.

The Relational Placebo

Humans have been variously described as the social animal and the language animal. It is thus understandable that the features common to traditional and contemporary analyses of placebos and nocebos, whatever the actual mechanisms postulated for their biological modes of action, are the centrality of words and signs and the caregivers who are responsible for their presentation. Physicians and the contexts in which they provide care are implicated in the childhood associative learning experiences that create the functional links between words and signs and the minds/bodies of persons who are later patients and subjects. Moreover, caregivers and contexts are then the source of the triggers that evoke the placebo responses in clinical and experimental encounters. The physician and the clinical context together provide an anticipatory framework for healing and the reduction of suffering by promising to reduce the uncertainty and fear of the unknown engendered by puzzling and threatening symptoms, by extending compassion and concern, and by offering the expertise that may hasten a renewed state of well-being.

Placebos achieve their effects within the physician–patient relationship and are initiated by the words and actions of the clinician operating on the experientially prepared mind/body of the patient. Balint, writing in 1952, described the physician as a drug—what a later author referred to as the doctor's "growing pharmacological awareness of self."[33] The placebo, though chemically inert, gains its power in part through the meanings implicit in the words and behaviors of the caregiver and the accompanying contextual cues, interacting with the patient's responses to the rituals of their interactions.

This understanding of placebos is reflected in comments from scholars in the field. Benedetti writes that "interactions between therapists and their patients trigger physiologic mechanisms that have so far been neglected."[34] Findley notes that "the physician is a vastly more important institution than the drug store."[35] Miller and colleagues, writing on interpersonal healing, state that "the communicative interaction of practitioners with patients, both verbal and nonverbal, may produce placebo effects even without the use of discrete treatments."[36] And, conversely, an "uninterested"[37] physician may undermine the effects of open-label placebos.

The beliefs of the placebo administrator influence the efficacy of the placebo response experienced by the patient. In a double-blind study of the treatment of pain following a dental extraction, Gracely and colleagues[38] told one group of clinicians administering the analgesic infusions that one group of patients would be randomized to receive either saline or naloxone and a second group might receive one of three possible infusions, namely saline, naloxone, or fentanyl, a potent analgesic. The reports of postoperative pain in the placebo arms of the two groups, each receiving saline infusions, were dramatically different—the first group reported an increase in pain whereas the second group reported a significant decrease in pain. Neither the subjects nor the clinicians were aware of the content of the actual infusion—yet, the belief by the clinicians attending the second group that some subjects may be receiving fentanyl was somehow inadvertently telegraphed to the subjects, thereby eliciting a placebo response. The anticipations of the placebo administrators as well as those of the subjects contribute to the placebo responses actually elicited.

The influence of placebo providers was demonstrated in a simulated clinical interaction in which the beliefs and expectations of providers could be experimentally manipulated.[39] Normal subjects were assigned to the roles of doctor or patient and participated in the experiment. In the first step, the doctors were conditioned to believe that a cream labeled "thermedol" was an analgesic by applying a lower temperature stimulus to the skin treated with thermedol and a higher temperature stimulus to a skin spot treated with a cream labeled "placebo." In reality and unbeknownst to the subjects, both creams were the same inert material. Once the subjects in this doctor group were successfully conditioned to the analgesic cream, thermedol, they were asked to treat the patients with thermedol or placebo and test the effects using the temperature stimuli. In this second step of treatment the temperature of the test skin probes were the same, namely, the high temperature, and the doctors were instructed to refrain from identifying the nature of the creams actually applied. In other words, they believed they were participating in a single-blind experiment in which they knew which cream was applied to their patients in each trial but were not permitted to reveal that information to their patients. In each of several replications, the patients reported less pain when the doctors believed they had applied thermedol compared with placebo cream. In addition to these verbal reports of less pain, the patients in these thermedol groups exhibited lower arousal as measured by skin conductance. By contrast, the patients in the placebo cream group reported greater pain, higher arousal, and more elements of facial expressions associated with pain. While the doctors' facial expressions did differ between the applications of thermedol and placebo, these differences did not account for the differential pain reactions of their patients. Thus, while the placebo effects were "socially transmitted" via what the authors describe as an "interpersonal expectancy effect," the actual signals or indicators by which the doctors transmitted their conditioned beliefs or expectations to their patients remain a mystery. Whatever the actual mode of signaling of information or expectations, the authors of this empirical study arrived at the same conclusions as Balint with their observation regarding "one of the oldest and most powerful medical treatments—healers themselves."[40]

Placebo Is Metaphor

The conceptual formulation by Balint of the doctor as drug suggests a metaphoric construct in which (some of) the pharmacologic properties of the drug are transferred to the doctor, leading to DOCTOR IS DRUG as the metaphor. This reflects the idea that (some of) the properties normally attributed to drugs, for example, pain relief or enhanced mood, are also properties of the doctor. This can be understood as an extended metaphor from the more general construction PLACEBO IS X, in which the X can be any clinical intervention—drugs, surgery, or any method with known pharmacological or physiological effects. The PLACEBO is an intervention, procedure, or substance, normally considered clinically inert that can be newly understood to demonstrate (some of) the clinical properties of the traditional intervention. The root metaphor PLACEBO IS X is compendious and accommodates a diverse array of extensions. Some are unexpected, for example, that sham surgery is effective in certain clinical situations, and sufficiently surprising to warrant publication in major medical journals and newspapers. Others, such as the doctor as placebo, are so engrained in our cultural understanding as to have become commonplace literal language. It is only by comparison to healing rituals from communities other than our own that we begin to appreciate the ritualistic power of our clinical practices. In fact, just as placebo responses in clinical trials have increased with the widespread use of medications for the exigencies of daily living, the actual growth in efficacy of contemporary medicine can heighten the placebo benefits of physicians. There is a considerable likelihood that ritual power will be attributed to big machines, impressive technologies, and the advent of medical robots and telemedicine. We may then need to relearn that, as is the case with pills and rituals, the healing potency is resident in the prescribing physician or performing shaman, that is, in the persons entwined in the clinical relationship.

In many metaphors the properties or connotations transferred are primarily cognitive, though some, for example, ARGUMENT IS WAR, are laden with emotional and affective impact, as a heated debate and a fight to the end. In the case of placebos, the connotations are both cognitive and affective and, as we have noted, the transferred connotations can be cryptic to both parties, yet the physiological power is evident in the responses and outcomes. This understanding can be broadened to encompassing words and signs as linguistic and semiotic placebos, at first seemingly inert, yet laden with enormous clinical potency that helps us perceive the entire placebo phenomenon as a pharmacology of words and signs. An additional insight from the metaphoric framing of placebos stems from the field of cognitive linguistics, which understands metaphors as evidence of neural networks and connectivities among representations of words and concepts that underlie seeing one thing in terms of another heretofore unrelated entity. The associations that underlie placebo responses may be no different than those that empower language. Placebos depend on previously learned connections, whether by conditioning or more subtle experiential linkages that create the readiness for the clinical responses. Hence, when the words and signs of the caregiver trigger physiological and neurochemical systems such as endogenous opioids, they are mediated by neural networks that connect cognitive, affective, and hormonal cascades in the brains/bodies of the patients. And, just as linguistic metaphors reshape how we see the worlds in which we live, placebos reframe how we entrain bodily responses in coping with illness.

Diamonds Are Forever

The entangled story of placebos, signs, and the power of inertness can be unknotted through a heuristically useful example—diamonds. These bits of compressed carbon are to the chemist perfect exemplars of inertness and to the engineer means of cutting and polishing other hard substances. By contrast, to the dealer in gemstones and the romantically inclined customers, diamonds are of enormous value, both monetary and sentimental. Diamonds adorn the crowns of royalty and the paraphernalia of sultans and sports stars. A gift of a diamond may signal an offer of matrimony or symbolize a lifelong commitment. The gem may evoke the tachycardia of anticipation and the autonomic facial blush of love and arousal. This inert substance is laden with meaning and symbolism created by social and cultural understandings shaped by enormously successful marketing over a period of a century and a half. And, as in the case of placebos, the cognitive and affective power of the diamond and its capacity to evoke mind/body responses depend intimately on the identity of the person offering the gift, the implicit intent, and the contextual cues of setting, lighting, music, words, and the like. The associative learning that sensitizes both parties is acquired in a cultural context with the relevant rituals rehearsed endlessly in well-crafted advertisements and a carefully regulated marketplace. Not only are diamonds excellent models of placebos that are chemically inert yet pharmacologically potent, they also represent open-label placebos that depend on overt expression for their power. Lastly, these gems also exemplify cultural and generational change that may undermine the long-celebrated slogan that "diamonds are forever." By contrast with former medical students who reacted to the word *diamond* with a response of romance, more recent generations are triggered to think of blood diamonds and servitude in the mines of southern Africa. Perhaps the potency of current formulations of placebos will also be reshaped by cultural evolution and become akin to the snake-oil potions of early nineteenth-century medical charlatans. Indeed, what may last forever are not diamonds and pills but the power of words and symbols.

IV

HEALING THE LANGUAGE AND THE LANGUAGE OF HEALING

11
The Physician–Patient Relationship

When Dr. Rabolinski showed up the next morning, Olive waited to see if he had heard of her horror, and when he did not mention it, she finally said, "My bowels moved with a frightful ferocity." She made herself look at him when she said that. He said, "It's the antibiotics," and gave a small shrug. So she relaxed a tiny bit and asked when she could go home, and he said, "Any day now." He sat on the bed after that, without saying anything, and Olive gazed out the window. For a few moments she felt something close to bliss, but it was more as though time had stopped—just for these few moments time had stopped—and there was only the doctor and life, and it sat with her in the morning sunshine that fell over the bed. She put her hand on his briefly, and still looking out the window she said, quietly, "Thank you," and he said, quietly, "You're welcome."

—Elizabeth Strout, *Olive Again*

The practice of medicine is enacted between a patient and a physician engaged in a clinical relationship that is mutually crafted. It is a particular genre of human interactions. Medical care, whether provided in a hospital, clinic, or the patient's home, is a response by the physician to an expressed desire or need by the patient for explanation, reassurance, clarification, or restoration. The patient–physician relationship differs from most human engagements in that one party is ill and perhaps vulnerable and seeks help, while the doctor possesses the capacities and skills to respond. This difference in capabilities adds to the obligations and duties of the clinician to respond to the request from the patient and engage fully and directly.

As is true of all human interactions, clinical engagement is enacted in words and language, both verbal and nonverbal. The gravity of the process and the import of its outcomes to both parties make the interchanges highly sensitive to the nuances of words, their meanings, and modes of expression. Whether we consider the stories that patients bring to the encounter, the diagnostic explanations proffered by the doctor, or the recommendations for remedies and reassurance—all these linguistic acts are highly modulated by and sensitive to meanings and metaphors.

Military tropes set up an adversarial interaction between the physician and the disease that is viewed as the prime object of medical attention. The language of alliance, by contrast, contemplates a consensual understanding between patient and physician of the goals of care so that even if disease is seen as the enemy to be fought, then, at the least, the caregiver and the person who is ill are allies and collaborators. Ideally, the alliance does not frame disease as an objectified enemy but rather a process of illness and an imbalance to be understood and rectified. In either instance, the collaborative framing renders the patient as the prime focus of the physician's attention and duty. The patient's illness and the person's unique rendition of its course are the clues for understanding, whereas the military metaphor ignores illness and attends exclusively to the adversarial disease. Similarly, diagnostics in the latter frame searches for clues to causal agents, while the collaborative approach seeks to decipher the patient's story to understand the genesis of the illness. The distinction between the two perspectives is more striking when considering therapeutics. The military metaphor demands conquest and extirpation of the disease, whereas attention to the patient perceives a need for relief and seeks a means of restoration.

The difference in emphasis between the military metaphor and the collaborative understanding extends beyond the instance of illness to the larger canvasses of prevention and public health. The military looks to external causal agents, and prevention entails keeping foreign influences at bay. It renders prevention as constructing barriers to entry of viruses and other external threats. At the same time, ecological susceptibilities and organismal imbalances are ignored. A case in point is the emphasis during the recent COVID pandemic on closing borders and quarantine while simple and effective behavioral adaptations of masks and handwashing were thought by many to be weak and effete. At the same time, significant susceptibility factors such as obesity, smoking, homelessness, and poverty are ignored as immaterial to the issue of public health. We also witnessed the debacle of considering public health as a set of reactive responses to the perfect storm of an epidemic, akin to a military response to a surprise invasion. Yet, the chaos of a pandemic stemmed not from unpredictable random events (in faraway lands) but were foreseen by experts and specialists as a highly probable occurrence. These warnings were pooh-poohed and ignored. Paradoxically, "war-game" exercises forecast the emergence of a serious respiratory viral infection, yet even the military mavens were cast aside in a fantasyland of strange and surreal optimism. This recent cataclysmic pandemic failed to evoke a national, let alone international, collaborative agreement to plan for, mitigate, and perhaps even avert the next global crisis, whether due to a virus, climate change, chronic global endemic illnesses, or shortages of affordable medications and vaccines.

The divergence in viewpoint between these two metaphors is reflected in many of the social responses to the pandemic that variously emphasized individual autonomy, at times at a cost to the health of others, and ignored the idea of the commonweal and the benefits of living in a community-embedded, relational environment. The impact of different metaphors on the categories of medical practice is evident in the action-oriented, military model of acute medicine, for example, surgery, trauma, and emergency medicine, compared with the incremental steps and patience on the part of both patients and physicians in adapting to and ameliorating the lives of persons with chronic illnesses. It is not surprising that fire engine medicine captures the imagination of the general public and Hollywood filmmakers, while caring for elderly persons with restrictions due to chronic illnesses are seen by many to constitute a societal burden. Language shapes our minds, frames our perspectives, and determines our actions, both for good and for ill.

The Missing Patient

A medical understanding rooted in the natural sciences has been traced by some to the social and pedagogical power of the 1910 Flexner Report to the Carnegie Foundation[1] with its critical observation that a major part of North American medical training was unregulated and highly variable in quality with curricula that were often undocumented or nonexistent. The report led to substantial reforms in medical education and the introduction of a foundational base of scientific knowledge in medical training. Massive government investment in biomedical research in the 1940s led to significant changes in the understanding of diseases and to improvements in pharmacological interventions and vaccines. These reforms and initiatives, and their ancillary benefits, reshaped medical schools and teaching hospitals and promoted a thorough enchantment with science and the desire to repair broken bodies. An unfortunate corollary of these large and important changes was the diminished attention to and presence of the patient in the medical cosmos.

Over the past forty years, physicians and medical educators have proposed a variety of novel schemas and frameworks designed to reintroduce the patient into the visual field of clinical attention. The intention was not to undermine the necessary rootedness of medical knowledge in the biomedical and natural sciences but to redirect the clinical gaze toward the patient. A realignment would bridge the growing divide between doctors and patients highlighted in Elliot Mishler's study of a clinical encounter.[2] The two participants resided in two non-intersecting worlds—the patient ensconced in a lifeworld of daily concerns inflected by an intercurrent illness, while the physician searches for the disease from within the world of medicine. The analysis underscored the growing concerns among both doctors and patients that an absence of coherent perspectives would result in misaligned objectives and goals. The idea was to recover those clinical skills directed to the patient as person rather than as the vessel or bearer of disease. These would include reminders of the duties of the profession to care for and about the patient and to understand the illness in order to diminish suffering, reduce uncertainty, and provide opportunities for support, trust, and hope.

In a 1977 paper in *Science*, entitled "The Need for a New Medical Model: A Challenge for Biomedicine," George Engel challenged the predominant medical model of the past two centuries of Western medicine as promulgated by the Paris school of early nineteenth-century France that viewed the physician as a clinical pathologist of the living body, just as the anatomical pathologist examined the body through biopsies or autopsies. The pathologist may understand the object of professional attention to be the disease construed in terms of cellular pathology and mutated genes. Engel argued that the object of study of the clinician is the human being who understands and presents the illness in narratives populated with biological, behavioral, and psychosocial information. The physician does not deal directly with the disease, nor with the body, but with the person, and the resultant imperative to comprehend the behavioral and psychosocial is simply because, to cite Engel, "these are the terms in which most clinical phenomena are reported by patients."[3] Engel's aim was to describe a clinical epistemology in which the object of knowledge for the clinician is the person and access to the circumstances of the illness can be gained and ascertained only with the patient, not simply by peering into the patient with an endoscope or through the patient via an MRI.

Michael Saraga and colleagues have analyzed the writings of Engel both in his early paper introducing the biopsychosocial model and in a later paper in *Psychosomatics*[4] and proposed that Engel's purpose was an epistemic reframing of clinical practice.[5] His goal was not in the first instance an insistence that etiological factors in illness should encompass psychosocial factors in addition to biological elements. Moreover, his innovative idea was not the admixture of a humane attitude on the part of the physician as a complement to a reductive scientific stance but rather a shift of epistemic emphasis from the disease to the patient. In so doing, the patient can no longer be a minor element at the periphery of the clinician's visual field, and the centrality of the patient becomes a matter for clinical skills and competence and not reliant solely on a moral obligation that can be ignored when inconvenient.

Regrettably, the elements of the biopsychosocial model that captured the attention of many contemporary colleagues were the result of a misplaced emphasis on the etiological and humane aspects of Engel's proposal that became the prime legacies of his model. That is, what medicine needs is a broader concept of etiology in which psychosocial factors would add to and perhaps balance the traditional list of causal factors well populated by infectious agents and carcinogenic chemicals. A second appealing aspect of that reading may have been the implicit addition of "elements of the humane, such as warmth, intimacy, solicitude and compassion"[6] to the tried and true clinical skills of percussion and auscultation and other aspects of physical diagnosis. The outcomes of these interpretations were two unfortunate dichotomies and dualities. The first insists that we must add, in some complex clinical calculus, elements of the psychological disposition of the patient and the social context of life to the more readily definable biological factors of risk and causality. That is, it is not the recognition that additional elements are relevant to the development of illnesses that is the source of our current dilemma, but rather the consideration that psychosocial and biological factors are somehow categorically different. It is as if illness results from an unfortunate admixture of elements of the biological when incubated in a maladapted psychological setting. Such models of additivity continue to reflect an old Cartesian distinction between the mind and body and make it difficult to appreciate the seamless continuity of psyche and soma and the embodiment of both persons and their illnesses.

The second duality that continues to resonate as a bicameral shadow over clinical practice is the split of the clinician into two personas so that the procedural skills and biomedical knowledge of the cold and calculating technician must be balanced or somehow softened by a humane alter-ego with the attitudes of caring, sensitivity, and compassion. The first set is described as technical skills and the second by character traits of personality. Again, we are confronted with a dichotomy and patients debate false choices between a surgeon who cuts and one who cares! Engel's attempt to avoid a reductionist understanding of disease was misread as a desire to broaden the etiological framework of causality and his insistence that the object of clinical study is the human was misconstrued as a need for a humane, as well as skilled, physician. As a result, both patients and physicians are sundered along their own fault lines: patients are susceptible to somehow separable biological and psychosocial causal factors, and physicians are exhorted to be both skilled and compassionate as if those were competing commitments.

The resultant dichotomies aligned with other well-worn dualities, including the science and art of medicine, the head and heart of the physician, and specialties that were construed as hard and technical or soft and touchy-feely. The understandable response to these unfortunate and unintended consequences of Engel's contribution was a series of proposals to heal the divisions and aim for a holistic or integrative model of care. Many of these frameworks acknowledged and accepted the dichotomies and recommended an oscillation between the dual mandates of the physician, of curing and caring. Or, as expressed in an early model of patient-centered medicine, the physician's task should be "twofold: to understand the patient and to understand the disease."[7] Some models fostered an integration between allopathic approaches and those of complementary and alternative medicine, and many made distinctions between doctor- and patient-centered medicine. Nonetheless, the underlying ethos of many such offerings retains the dual discourse that, by its very presence, undermines a functional understanding of the relationship between physicians and patients and their entwined duties and roles that enable the goals of clinical care.

Perhaps the best-known and most commonly cited concept in the effort to reform medical education and health care is "patient-centeredness" that metaphorically places the ill person at the focal point of medical attention. The notion that the patient's concerns must be uppermost in the mind of the physician is an important reminder of the clinician's obligations. Yet, a metaphoric centrality implies a figurative structure at whose center is the patient. This brings to mind the well of an amphitheater with the patient surrounded by consultants and their eager trainees, a common trope in traditional artistic depictions of medical and surgical education in Europe and North America. Or, in later renditions, a patient in a hospital bed surrounded by an attending physician and a ward team on clinical rounds. Perhaps, more contemporaneously, the patient as digital image is at the center of a computer screen being viewed by an internist or in the lens of a surgical robot being manipulated by a distant surgeon.

The patient is undoubtedly the center of attention, but, sadly and all too often, appears alone and lonely and as an object that is seen rather than a subject who is heard or a partner who is engaged. These images, both real and figurative, reflect and underwrite another dichotomy or division, that is, between patient and physician. Rather than showing both parties joined in the clinical task, the patient is thrust into the center by the physician who is permitted to remain at the periphery. This affords a certain distancing effect that is experienced by the clinician as needed detachment, but the patient feels isolated. The effect is contrary to Michael Balint's pithy description of the clinical relationship as "a mutual investment company"[8]—a joint commitment to a long-term undertaking designed to provide benefits to both parties—healing for the patient and the fulfilment of a duty for the physician. This entanglement of roles is reflected during all medical visits. While the patient may be the sole author of the early story of illness, the clinical narrative is necessarily co-constructed with the physician and the trajectory of illness is a jointly authored and crafted work. We often refer to the medical interview with the phrase "taking the history." Perhaps a more accurate descriptor would be creating the history, or better still, co-creating the history of illness. As those who study history attest, history is not discovered but invented in retrospect.

The patient-centered method was certainly not introduced to separate physicians and patients, yet the implicit metaphor had consequences completely unintended and contrary to the outcomes desired by the innovators. This divisive effect is even more evident in later models that added new dimensions to the original construct, foremost among them patient autonomy, empowerment, and patient-directed care. While these differ from one another in several respects, they share a common feature of affording an increasing degree of independence of action for patients in gauging the clinical issues, selecting those of greatest concern to their own well-being, and making their own decisions by choosing among the options for interventions and management. These frameworks are natural extensions of the idea of patient-centered medicine spurred by understandable responses to long traditions of paternalistic health care by a male-dominated profession. Comprehending and respecting the sensibilities, concerns, and needs of patients by placing them at the center of the clinical agenda are necessary elements of effective health care that considers the dignity of patients as persons. However, once again, the metaphoric entailments of these concepts have generated effects not foreseen by those who promulgated their introduction.

Calling for autonomy and empowerment for patients signals increased concerns for personhood, dignity, and respect for persons who are ill. They serve to balance regimes in which the needs and desires of patients are ignored by an authoritarian, perhaps militaristic cadre of doctors. However, the proposed solutions are fraught with risks and unanticipated effects. The consequences are explored by the ethnographer Annmarie Mol in her book, *The Logic of Care: Health and the Problem of Patient Choice,* in which she compares two guiding regimes, the logic of choice and the logic of care. The former endorses patient autonomy and is based on the presumption that we are all autonomous individuals, leading to the view that "autonomy and equality are good and oppression is bad."[9] By contrast, the logic of care understands that "attentiveness and specificity are good and neglect is bad." The author reminds us that "when ... patients complain about bad health care, they may mention that they were not given a choice, but more often they talk about neglect. They describe how their particular stories or personal experiences were not attended to."[10] Patients do not seek a physician who makes them feel empowered and autonomous but rather singled out as unique, significant, and worthy of attention. Independence of choice and action are not their desiderata of clinical care; instead of autonomy, patients desire an attunement "to people who are first and foremost related."[11] They seek a bond with their caregivers. Mol points out that a societal and perhaps professional failure to describe and promulgate notions of good care left a space for the advent of autonomy and empowerment as poor substitutes. More cogently, she observes that "the logic of choice ... can shift the weight of everything that goes wrong to the shoulders of the patient-chooser."[12]

The conclusion that an emphasis on autonomy and empowerment can have the perverse side effects of blame and guilt is echoed in the work of the health psychologists Peter Salmon and Bridget Young in their studies of patients in an oncology clinic. They find that patients do not seek control or choice and that illness itself reduces the need, desire, and capacity to make independent choices. Patients seek information from clinicians not for purposes of making decisions but as a means of building rapport and trust in the relationship and maintaining hope for the future. They seek the physician's expertise and value options more than choices; patients do not wish to feel overwhelmed with information. Autonomy lies not in the right to make choices but in being informed about the choices considered and made by clinicians whose expertise patients trust. This provides a needed sense of safety and confidence in plans for treatment and interventions. In that sense and perhaps somewhat paradoxically, "autonomy is relational."[13] Patients have opinions and wish to be acknowledged and heard; they do not necessarily express a need to make their own decisions and choices.

Salmon and Hall[14] express additional concerns about asking patients to be involved in decisions regarding care associated with undue expectations of agency and responsibility for their own well-being. Physicians are thereby permitted to diminish their own engagement and assume fewer obligations to attend to difficult and demanding situations for which simple treatment options are not readily available. These commonly include unrelenting pain, existential suffering, and chronic conditions for which cures are rare but patient and persistent care remains paramount. Obscure illnesses and medically unexplained symptoms may lead to the displacement of responsibility to the patient. When treatable disease is not evident, physicians feel unable to help and patient-centeredness may become not a mode of sharing control but a means of shifting responsibility and assigning blame. The authors describe discussions between physicians and patients with chronic, unexplained symptoms in which each tries to draw the other in a tug of war toward grounds on which each can cast aspersions on the other. The physician might declare that medicine has nothing to offer for imaginary pains and the patient might retort that the physician does not care to grasp the suffering and angst. In consequence, medicine withdraws, and patients are left to fend for themselves—so much for autonomy! Once patients are empowered, or burdened, with control of treatment decisions, they have only themselves to blame should things go awry. Ironically, persons suffering chronic illness with unexplained symptoms are apt to judge their physicians by their abilities to form and maintain alliances with their patients and not by the absence of successful diagnoses and treatments.

Salmon and Hall[15] emphasize the consequences of undue burdens placed on patients by pointing to the war language that continues to inflect the discourse in the clinic, especially in oncology care. The admonitions of caregivers to their patients to fight, stay positive and optimistic and persistent may be well intended to buoy the spirits and empower persons coping with the demands of illness. However, these efforts better serve the needs of the physicians to remain hopeful and do not help the sufferers. Patients respond by adapting their behaviors to alleviate burdens on their family members and clinicians and thereby suppress their own expressions of suffering. After all, fighting entails keeping a stiff upper lip and not revealing self-doubts and fear of failure. Thus, employing the language of war to empower patients may in fact undermine those who need to be supported by thoughtful concern and compassionate attentiveness and permitted to articulate their own fears and doubts.

Teams and JAMS

A related phenomenon was described by Balint, with the phrase "a collusion of anonymity."[16] Patients with challenging problems may be attended by multiple specialists and consultants, each offering helpful suggestions and advice. The necessarily complex management plan and vital decisions are adopted with no identifiable person assuming responsibility. In addition, questions from the ill person and family are redirected from one clinician to another but never clarified to the satisfaction of the puzzled patient. When responsibility is diffused, no single person takes on the role of team leader or becomes clearly identified as such to the patient who may have questions and concerns. Patients also report a similar situation when an extensive health care team of physicians, nurses, and allied health professionals contributes different aspects of the clinical care and, after bedside rounds, exits the hospital room en masse, leaving the patient to worry and wonder in isolation. As an aside, medical students are familiar with such scenarios of bevies of consultants and teams of caregivers coming and going while the young trainees present in the hospital often become identified by the patient as "my doctor." They are often the recurrent and regularly available and identifiable person who actually sits at the bedside and listens. As a result, medical students suffer from the JAMS syndrome—Just a Medical Student—as in, there was nothing I could do, so I just sat and spent time with the patient. Students thereby learn that listening to patients is not central to clinical care, even as they are burdened with questions from patients that they are yet ill equipped to address. The young trainees become caught—between the pride in being acknowledged by patients as a valued member of a health care team and the paradoxical behavior of role models who demonstrate that spending time with patients is unimportant.

The Framework of Relationships

Researchers trying to understand the needs and desires of patients discover that persons with illness express both a desire and a need to be in a dyadic partnership with a caregiver who understands and enacts the duty of care. In a qualitative study of clinical care, John Scott and colleagues[17] elicited the experiences of patients and physicians and identified three important elements of a functioning dyadic relationship. Relational care contributes to what both patients and physicians characterize as healing and are summarized by those elements. Trust is described as a sense of feeling cared for, the knowledge that promises will be kept, and a needed safe space within which the patient may feel vulnerable yet protected. The second is hope, a state of belief that there can be a positive future beyond the present state of suffering and uncertainty. Not a facile promise that all will be well but rather a sense that the caregiver retains a commitment to work diligently such that all may be well once again. Or, more modestly, that hope resides in the small joys of the day-to-day, not necessarily in a far distant future. Third is a sense of being known, a genuine feeling that the caregiver knows the patient and all that is significant to that person as an individual. Moreover, the patient learns that the clinician is invested in that individual's welfare, demonstrable by the recognition that the patient and physician appreciate and enjoy a shared history and a consensus of concerns and hopes for a future. Such relational outcomes are associated with improved quality of patients' lives; they correlate with better clinical outcomes and have the ancillary benefit of enriching the daily lives of clinicians.

The need for a relational understanding is expressed in stronger terms by patients with medically unexplained symptoms. Their common experiences of having been ignored or viewed as demanding lead to a keen desire for a partnership with a clinician who is willing to engage in a conversation and thereby exhibit a genuine interest in the patient's symptoms and the context of the specific personal circumstances. Such persons seek a caregiver who is capable of listening to the patient's constructs of causality, has the patience to elicit and assuage underlying fears and anxieties, and can validate the suffering and angst. In a word, the patient gains the sense of being taken seriously within an authentic relationship.

Many clinicians learn and adopt practical and simple actions that create and nurture a clinical relationship. Recognizing the individuality of the patient is evident in ordinary yet important elements of all authentic communication, including eye contact, smiling, and speaking in a modulated voice rather than a monotone. One thoughtful approach is to make the patient feel unique and special, for example, complimenting the person's demeanor or resilience. Most helpful is to spend a few minutes speaking about something of interest to the patient but unrelated to the disease or treatment. The patient's individuality can also be acknowledged by a clinician who is somewhat informal, by using humor or simply considering the patient as a full persona rather than the object of treatment. One small, though telling, suggestion is to have important discussions with patients once they are fully dressed and not disrobed on the examination table. Respect for the patient is also communicated by simple yet important cues, for example, avoiding technical terms and acronyms and using concepts and tropes that are familiar to that individual. Again, the notion of patient choice is not an issue of actual selection among treatment options. Patients state that identifying appropriate management is the job of the physician; however, what they value is being informed, that is, the opportunity to concur. It is quite striking and perhaps telling that patients view a clinician who takes the time to sit, listen, and provide reassurance as a departure from the expected and how much that is valued as emblematic of a genuine relationship. A potent, authentic, simple, and clinical mode of language, both verbal and behavioral, was deftly captured by Mol: we need "a language in which the main emphasis is not on autonomy and right to decide for oneself, but on daily life practices and attempts to make these more livable through inventive doctoring."[18]

Clinical Presence

The relational model of care is predicated on the interactions between physicians and patients and understands clinical practice as a dyadic activity between two individuals that implements the process of caring for the needs of the person with illness. The role and behavior of the physician in the arena of care has been termed "clinical presence," defined by a group of researchers in a series of qualitative studies at Stanford University as "a purposeful practice of awareness, focus, and attention with the intent to understand and connect with individuals/patients."[19] These enactments are thoughtful actions by physicians with the goal of deepening the connections with patients in the situation of clinical care. Physicians are responsible for these practices, but they are directed to benefit their patients in the relational dyad. Clinical presence includes attention to physical presence, being there with intent as opposed to a harried visit. The arrangement of chairs and persons, and whether the space is organized to promote egalitarian eye contact, warrants notice. Space includes the "metaphorical ... space for the unknown" while, as the authors observe, "clinicians aren't comfortable with the unknown."[20] Good clinicians are cognizant of other physical intrusions, including cell phones, computers, and email and are intent to avert such distractions. The actual ritual of the clinical visit, whether in the hospital or office, is important in connoting the healing power that patients associate with the physician. Handwashing, demeanor, and a quiet environment help set the tone, and special attention to the temporal quality of presence is relevant. An attentive physician is perceived by patients as being present longer than one who remains in the room for an equivalent period but telegraphs a sense of haste and competing priorities. Time also has an intangible dimension, described by one observer as "intense connected moment(s)."[21]

The encounter between a patient and doctor can be a very short, one-time interaction in a walk-in clinic or an emergency department, generally for a specific, immediate need. At the other end of the time spectrum are primary care physicians who have ministered to two or more generations of a family and enjoy a decades-long relationship with the patients in care. Whether an isolated event or a lifelong association, the need for careful and engaged attention is ever-present. One may even argue that the rapid assessment and demand for quick decisions add a particular urgency and intensity to the staccato encounter in the trauma center. Of course, the nature of the clinical relationship that may evolve in the care of a patient with a chronic, serious illness will enhance the physician's familiarity with the lifeworld of the patient and the access to hidden concerns and cryptic metaphors. Thus, clinical relationships have variable timelines of face-to-face encounters; however, whether short-lived or lifelong, the demand to be present and respond to the specific needs of the person asking for care remains constant. And the relationship exists and continues beyond and between the actual clinical encounters. A patient may recall and reflect on the physician's words long after leaving the clinic or hospital and those recollections may be a source of comforting solace or anxious concern. The physician may review X-rays and laboratory data or consult with colleagues regarding a specific patient in preparation for a visit or prior to an operation. Thus, like many human associations, clinical relationships proceed episodically, yet may also evolve continuously.

Presence is a means to achieve a sense of connectedness between patients and physicians that is fostered by a clinician prepared to pause and receive a patient's story. The goal of listening in this setting is not to respond but to understand and create a bond by demonstrating the desire to appreciate the narrative and witness the suffering and angst. The focus is on the present moment in time and not on what must be done tomorrow or next week. Presence is inherent in the value of being there for its own sake and not necessarily for some other instrumental goal.

Once the initial overtures toward connectedness lead to a burgeoning sense of trust, the relational space may enlarge to permit a process of joint, rather than solipsistic, reflection between patient and physician. The process of attentive listening in silence will have provided access to the concerns, needs, and fears of the patient. Joint consideration begins to craft a consensual agenda for action beyond the present moment, which in turn provides a scaffold and a process for informed, sensitive decisions and clinical actions to implement care and engender healing.

The importance of the relationship is evident in the results of a literature review conducted by Friedrich Stiefel and Céline Bourquin to identify factors that foster communications skills in trainees in oncology. They note that decision-making depends on relational engagement that instills a sense of trust in patients and affords an authentic human connection with clinicians. This interaction was described as a "nuanced dance," in which "trust outweighed the need for information"[22] and an "emotional relationship [that] did not require overt emotional talk"[23] but rather qualities such as expertise and authenticity. Indeed, clinicians' expertise and genuine engagement appear to be more valued by patients than expressions of compassion and sadness. The authors conclude that the relevant factors are the clinician's flexibility, a capacity to adapt to the singular patient, clinical imagination, and a sensitivity to the interactional aspects of communication. By contrast, it is evident that many programs designed to teach these clinical skills are actually Skinnerian training exercises to inculcate basic procedural skills by behavior modification. These programs are at best superficial. A clinician capable of relational engagement requires extended education through clinical experience in an apprenticeship with thoughtful and reflective role models. The process is not simply one of learning new skills but rather becoming a different person through formative experiences.

The dyadic relationship permits the clinical interaction to move beyond what is termed "taking a history of the illness" toward what Balint called a "deeper diagnosis." By listening to the patient's story, the physician learns and vicariously experiences the patient's world and gains a sense of that person's lived reality, both prior to and during illness. A series of such joint reflections will also provide access to the patient's hopes and desires for both present and future—all relevant to the clinician's pragmatic work of offering diagnostic insights and appropriate therapies. The framing concept is not empathy in the sense of stepping into the patient's shoes but that of a curious and committed participant-observer on a field trip to the land of the ill. This is not the visit of a tourist but the mission of a duty-bound physician.

The ethnographic trope developed by Engel in his understanding of the clinical interaction also reflects the relational aspect of these encounters. He describes the patient "as both an initiator and collaborator in the process" and the physician as "a participant observer" who attends to the "patient's reporting of inner-world data" and compares these with the clinician's "own personal inner viewing system for comparison and clarification."[24] The medium of this dialogic reflection is language and the process is described by Engel as "communing (sharing experiences)" and "communicating (exchanging information)." The method of clinical study is both *of* the patient and *with* the patient, providing access to the illness while "rendering patient data scientific."[25] Thus, the relational and dialogic framework eliminates the separation between patient and physician and avoids the parallel tracks and sundered links between the human and the scientific. The clinical perspective and necessary data can be gained only in partnership with the person who is ill. There is no disease separable from the ill patient and biological causality must be viewed in context of the psychosocial. As summarized by Saraga and colleagues, "Because the clinician is never dealing directly with a body but with a person, the 'disease-centered' or 'doctor-centered' approaches to the patient are simply illusory. There is no shortcut to gaining access to the disease: one gets there with the patient, not through the patient."[26]

Testimonies to the Relational

A series of wide-ranging interviews by Saraga and colleagues with experienced clinicians[27] and with patients[28] with chronic, serious illnesses yielded rich reflective descriptions of the lived realities of the clinical relationship from both perspectives. The summative term *engagement* encapsulates the physicians' testimonies and captures the "unitary lived experience of clinical practice."[29] Engagement underscores the relationship with the patient and entwines clinical practice, the person of the clinician, and the clinician's situation. The clinical situation exists because of the patient but extends beyond the physician–patient dyad to encompass all the elements that inflect the clinician's considerations and actions. These include colleagues, contexts, procedures and interventions with their guidelines and indications, and the physical artifacts of care, such as electronic records, surgical robots, and the enculturated understandings of the specific clinical environment. The situation includes the physician's inner landscape shaped by mentors, role models, and memorable clinical experiences, both happy and unfortunate, that accumulate and sediment to form an identity of norms and metrics that shape clinical judgments.

Engagement is witnessed in the specific and quotidian acts of clinical care. It refers to an individual physician, a specific patient, and a given setting. It extends in time for an entire trajectory of care that may be as short as a few minutes or as long as several years. The physician's engagement is continual in that it does not cease completely between visits but may encompass dealing with consultants, preparing for visits or perusing the published literature in seeking newer concepts of care. It may be evident in the commitment of an obstetrician who reorganizes a weekend call schedule in order to attend a woman in labor and in the late-night phone calls by a surgeon to the recovery room for a postoperative check on a certain patient. The specificity of engagement may seem daunting yet can also be reassuring in that the demand is not to know the patient in exhaustive detail but rather in the depth required in the given situation.

Engagement is parsed into its component features: doing an honest job, trespassing boundaries, creating a magic bubble, personal responsibility, and readiness. The first stems from the fact that daily clinical work is not heroic but must conform to standards of quality and care. It must be clear in its commitment to the duties of the physician and be carried out with diligence and punctiliousness. Good work demands perseverance and an attention to small details that may loom large in impact. Being meticulous and available were two common descriptors of quality cited by clinicians. When carried out well, honest work engenders trust and is characterized by seriousness of purpose and a modicum of obsessiveness and conscientiousness rather than flamboyance. One physician noted that "problems arise" not for "lack of brilliance, but ... things falling through the cracks."[30]

The second aspect of engagement that characterizes the relational nature of practice is described as trespassing boundaries. As one interviewee noted, "you do what you have to do,"[31] that is, what the clinical situation requires even if that entails breaking accepted rules of conduct. Given that many physicians regard their patients as members of their families, it is understandable that breaching boundaries becomes a minor evil if the specific setting requires actions against the grain. At times, doing an honest job may lead to an idiosyncratic clinical judgment that trumps an expected norm in order to accomplish the desired outcome. These are not the reflections of renegade or hot-headed physicians—these are clinicians with a deep sense of duty to the patient and strong commitments to their work.

Creating the magic bubble stems from a phrase used by a physician to describe an intimate moment in space and time enveloping the patient and physician to the exclusion of all else. This intense relational focus affords "a brief moment of connection where 'I have them and they have me.'"[32] Such protected spatiotemporal cocoons are not spontaneous occurrences but are intentionally created by masterly clinicians in the midst of a busy ward or emergency room to provide the space for "connexions"[33] and the relational bond.

Personal responsibility refers to a seriously felt sense of duty and obligation to the mandate and mission of practice. It includes doing an honest job and (paradoxically) breaching boundaries but extends to accepting personal responsibility when things turn out other than anticipated. It entails a capacity for self-critical reflection and a willingness to judge fairly. The responsibility includes "a sense of ownership not only of one's actions, but also of one's patients."[34] The expression indicates not that the physician owns the patients as a proprietary notion but rather takes on responsibility in a protective duty of care.

The last aspect, readiness, is, like personal responsibility, not a matter of enactment but an attitude or stance that characterizes the relational clinician. It describes a willingness to be engaged and a capacity of being open to the world of patients and their needs. It can suggest an eagerness for clinical interactions linked to a duty to respond to the call of the other and connotes a "disposition to stop and turn around."[35] Readiness incorporates a willingness and capability to accept a diverse set of inputs and symbols—listening in a broadened sense—that include the patient's demeanor, language, time and day of visit, and outcomes of prior consults and visits. It also implies an ability to set aside biases and prior conceptions that may impair a clear receptivity to the variety of signs from the individual seeking care.

The patient in a clinical relationship is similarly engaged in a clinical situation that encompasses the illness, the physician, the setting of care, and all the many factors that shape the cognitive and affective dimensions of being ill. These include family members, prior memories of symptoms and illnesses, previous interactions with caregivers, whether directly or vicariously, and the fears and uncertainties that color the inner landscape of the patient.

The experiences of patients with chronic, serious illnesses were explored in a set of extended interviews with cooperative volunteers. Three themes emerge from a detailed study of the transcripts of the patients' experiences of illness. These are the "shock on the realization of the illness, the chaos of the health care environment, and the anchor point provided by an engaged physician."[36]

The patient's sudden awareness of the advent of serious illness comes as a brutal break in the course and patterns of daily life. The life story is abruptly altered and the dream and vision for the future are clouded and uncertain. At times, the shock is induced by a worrisome symptom but more often by a single diagnostic word from a physician that makes quotidian worries fade into the background noise to be replaced by an overwhelming angst and awareness that life is inevitably and forever altered. Even harbingers that may turn out to be less than catastrophic, for example, minor lapses of memory, may be misread as the onset of early dementia and thereby evoke an awareness of a failing mind in a frail body. One patient was "stunned"[37] to find that a resident whom he met in a transplant clinic knew little of his medical history and his particularly complex clinical situation. Another patient with a lymphoma, himself a senior administrator of the institution in which he was receiving care, was "shocked" that the treating oncologist did not see fit to include the patient's wife in the discussions regarding treatment and was dismayed at entrusting his care to a seemingly uncaring physician.

Caregivers are insufficiently aware of the accounts and experiences of chaos that are the lived realities of patients who enter through what are to them the forbidding portals of hospitals, clinics, and the health care system more generally. Patients describe a confusing and unresponsive array of personnel and services. It is puzzling that in the midst of a system overflowing with data, forms, and computers patients remain uninformed regarding the persons responsible for their care, the plans for tests, and interventions, and often lack any inklings of the team's understanding of the patient's illness. One patient spoke of the hospital environment and her responses as follows: "It's chaotic. When students ask me, when they pose the question: 'But how is it? Really?'—this is chaos, you're entering into chaos."[38] The result of this doubled uncertainty—that is, the unknown nature of the illness and a lack of understanding of what the clinicians are thinking—is an abiding feeling of fear and lurking danger. The latter stems from examples of decisions taken quickly and perhaps in the absence of clear communication of important elements among members of a complex team of providers. To these are added instances of errors in medications, lost appointments, and forgotten promises. One patient related her confusion and dismay after arriving for consultations to which she had been referred: "I got myself there and they didn't even know why I was there. . . . I got myself there two or three times for nothing. They would look at me, and tell me: 'I don't know why you're here, I can't examine you.'" She concluded, "So, if I have a problem, there's no one in that hospital for me."[39] The patient's concern is not simply that the system is lax or inefficient but that the chaos may prove dangerous and even life-threatening. Little wonder then that "the participants experience the health care environment as unresponsive and absurd, to a degree reminiscent of the worlds of Franz Kafka and Lewis Carroll."[40]

Added to this feeling of risk and confusion that recalls the chaos narrative described by Arthur Frank is a corollary fear of being viewed as overly demanding or aggressive by asking too many questions and demanding answers and clarifications. Patients are keenly aware of their dependence for their welfare on their caregivers and experience what the investigators describe as "walking on eggshells."[41] They may unfortunately and inadvertently be placed in the role of supplicants rather than partners in the clinical relationship.

It is not surprising, therefore, that in the midst of feelings of shock and chaos, patients seek from their physicians a safe harbor and a sense of connection and security; what one patient called "an anchor point"—a connection with the clinician that engendered trust and turned the hospital from a setting of chaos to an oasis of respite and safety. For one patient who experienced this connection with a specific clinician, the feelings of chaos began to abate: "the hospital was my chalet—I went to the hospital for respite. It was a safe place for me despite the infections and the missed medication."[42] When this person was admitted to the hospital for care, she immediately requested that this particular clinician be advised. "I remember that he was really my anchor point, it was he, the person I trusted—that I trusted most in the world at that moment. When I talked to him, I had such a trust in that man, for everything."[43]

The anchor point for patients is constituted by the behavior and attitude of the clinician, and many elements contribute to this important sense of trust and safety for the patient. Perhaps the most important is the realization by the patient that the physician is working hard to understand the particular situation of the patient and is doing the job needed to respond to the implicit demand. In brief, it is the physician's engagement in the situation that constitutes the anchor point for the patient. Such engagement is made clear by evidence of a shared understanding of the fears and uncertainties with which the patient must contend and, furthermore, a shared concern for and sense of the desired outcome. A constant stance of listening to the patient coupled with a willingness to acknowledge the chaos and fears demonstrate that the physician is not only working hard but also able to reveal the worrisome concerns that accompany diligence and duty. Patients do not seek warmth and empathy as superficial expressions of emotion; rather, caring for the patient as a person is important as an index and incentive for perseverance and unrelenting concern. In brief, the opposite of detachment is not warmth but an abundance of engagement and depth of effort and care and the demonstrated commitment to do the best possible.

The patient and physician are thus each engaged in situations that are not congruent but complementary; they are not identical but relationally entwined. The patient is necessarily engaged by virtue of the illness and, ideally, elicits a response from a willing clinician. The physician's readiness describes the willingness to respond and engage. Yet, the clinician's engagement is not assured nor taken for granted but needs to be demonstrated. The patient seeks evidence of the authenticity and depth of the physician's engagement that signals that "we're in this together" coupled with the capability to accept responsibility and do an honest job. It is this clinical stance and subsequent work that generate trust and create the anchor point and safe harbor sought by the patient. The complementary, bilateral engagement constitutes the physician–patient relationship that provides the space for mutuality and the possibilities for healing.

The complementary engagements can also be described as bilaterally maieutic and mutually constitutive. The ill patient is ab initio engaged in a situation, but that does not per se connote clinical practice until a clinician responds to the call for help. Thus, there is no situation for the clinician without an engaged patient as midwife for the physician's engagement. Conversely, the physician's readiness and engagement are species and indicators of listening, thus enabling the narrative and testimony of the engaged patient. More than listening, it is the readiness to engage and do all that is required to provide care that enables the actions the patient seeks. The clinician who is willing to work honestly and diligently, who will break the rules if necessary and is ready to assume responsibility for care—these are the characterological attributes that create the magic bubble and protected space that provides the anchor point in a safe harbor. The anchor point is the individual clinician and the safe harbor is the reimagined setting for care. These actions support the patient in the journey through the shock and chaos and permit the co-creation of a healing relationship. Thus, the clinical relationship is not only an entwinement of the two complementary situations, it is itself constituted by the bilateral elicitation and responsiveness to the other. We cede the last word to a patient who observed, "A good physician would be someone who uses his knowledge and experience with the aim of supporting the patients. He supports them on their path. It is not a knowledge that you have innately, that you are using to show that you know things—it is to support and help the patients. A good physician for me respects his own humanity and respects his patients' humanity."[44]

12
Healing Metaphors

To most physicians, my illness is a routine incident in their rounds, while for me it's the crisis of my life. I would feel better if I had a doctor who, at least, perceived this incongruity.... I wouldn't demand a lot of my doctor's time; I just wish he would brood on my situation for perhaps five minutes, that he would give me his whole mind just once. I would like to think of him as going through my character, as he goes through my flesh, to get at my illness, for each man is ill in his own way.

—Anatole Broyard, (*Doctor, Talk to Me*)[1]

Clinicians as individuals and patients as individuals engage in a relational duet to achieve their mutual aims. The patient seeks explanations and wishes to understand the meaning and import of symptoms and signs. The patient also benefits from the comfort and reassurance that are secured within the safe haven offered by a trusted physician. The physician fulfills these significant clinical obligations by providing the requisite skills and expertise, exhibiting the calm authority to meet the patient's needs, while exercising the necessary modesty to refrain from unilaterally deciding what those may be. All the actions that follow—deciphering the patient's story, developing a mutual understanding of the nature of the illness, proceeding to selected examinations and tests, and jointly formulating and providing the appropriate therapeutic interventions—unfold within the dyadic context of the relationship created at the outset and deepened along the way. The joint understanding reached by consensus and the process of its attainment have been described as "a shared mind."[2]

The imperative for a clinical method that envisages each person/patient as unique was starkly evident in the recent pandemic. While many persons were infected with the virus that leads to COVID, the remarkable array of outcomes that resulted ranged from persons with few or no symptoms to patients requiring intensive care and mechanical ventilation. The diversity was seen even after infection by the precisely identical viral strain and among persons of the same age and pre-existing conditions. The pandemic was a dramatic example that while the "disease" may be the same, with all cases recorded and classified as COVID, the patients and their course of illness varied radically. This example highlights the fact that looking after a patient entails learning and responding to the specific request for care by that individual, at a given point in time. What provides relief and comfort for a sick person may change day to day and certainly varies with different stages of a specific ailment. The patient's feelings of chaos and fears of the unknown can be mitigated by the people that constitute the lived environment of family, friends, and colleagues. The objects and spaces of home, clinic, and hospital can influence the individual's physical and social contexts. Clinical practice, that is, caring for persons who are ill, is an engagement no less customized than the craft of the bespoke tailor and dressmaker who provide tailored garments and dedicated service. The proper practice of medicine does not flourish in a ready-to-wear environment and cannot be offered with a one-size-fits-all mindset. Medicine is thus not in pursuit of an ethical notion of a generally desired good that is, in any case, too general and nonspecific to serve as a guide. Medicine relies on a jointly constructed agreement and a deeply appreciative mutuality on the meanings of the illness and the actual needs and desires of the patient; thus, the good is specific and patient-dependent. While there is certainly an underlying, albeit fuzzy, moral imperative to do good and avert harm, a specific articulation of what constitutes good for the ill person and how to achieve that desired state exceeds the basic moral obligation and necessarily invokes the skills and experience of the engaged clinician.

An epidemiologist or public health physician is concerned with the characteristics of groups of persons and their averages, medians, variances, and distributions, providing knowledge of great value to the clinician. The latter is concerned, however, with the nature of the individual who is the patient and what that person requires at a given moment in time. The demand for specificity adds a dimension to the clinical skill of listening, as the clinician observer must receive the patient's story and concurrently determine the narrator's identity and concerns as they change with time and situation. These two sets of information, that is, the nature of the person who is ill and the evolving story of the illness, permit the clinician to engage in a mode of responsive communication that is adapted to the character and situation of the patient. The physician must use a mode of discourse that is clear and readily understood by the patient, and craft answers, provide information, and offer interpretations that are responsive to the expressed and, at times, unspoken concerns of the individual. Receiving and appreciating the lived experience of the narrator sets the stage for the tailored interactions and negotiations between a patient and a physician who can adapt the clinical presence to the values and preferences of the person. This flexibility will permit the calibrated sharing of information, interpretation, decision-making authority and power as well as the nuanced offerings of support, reassurance, and comfort. The mitigation of fear and uncertainty that attend the chaos of illness demands not a general offer of compassion or empathy. Rather, it requires intuition gained through the acquired skills of experience that offers an authentic sense to the patient that the physician is fully receptive, engaged, responsive, committed, and focused on the unique fears and deepest concerns of that patient.

The shared goal of the two persons in the clinical encounter is to collaborate in a process of healing. The word *healer* to describe a physician fell out of favor in the 1920s in America because of its association with shady characters peddling potions, charms, and illicit, sometimes toxic, remedies uncontrolled by any regulation and oversight. Healing was also regarded as antithetical to scientific medicine and best ascribed to shamans.

Healing offers a more expansive benefit than curing or caring can provide. The *Oxford English Dictionary* defines healing as a "restoration of wholeness, well-being, safety,"[3] and offers one definition of a physician as a "healer ... who cures moral, spiritual, or political ills."[4] The descriptions of becoming whole and feeling safe are important contrasts and responses to expressions of shock, chaos, and uncertainty, and the relief of existential and spiritual angst may achieve an important sense of feeling at home, reminding us of the medical chalet and the safe harbor sought by patients with serious illness. Chronic illness may be accompanied by disconnection from a social network, a deepening sense of vulnerability, failures of reasoning and memory, and the angst of loneliness and loss of purpose. These aspects of suffering are more usefully addressed within an expansive framework of healing of illness rather than the narrow perspective of curing a disease or that of caring, a word that has lost its traditional power.

Curing, understood as a return to a pristine a priori state, while desirable, is rare and too lofty a goal in many instances. It is too often a promise that is difficult to fulfill. Healing, by contrast, described as an increase in the well-being of the patient and, more specifically, improvement in the individual's functional capabilities to permit the patient to pursue the personal purposes of living, can serve as a touchstone for all medical care. Healing and curing are not necessarily aligned. Cures can be effected while angst remains. Physical pain can be relieved, yet suffering is unabated. Conversely, palliative care physicians describe patients whose disease was deemed incurable by oncologists with a comment that there is nothing more we can do, yet whose daily lives are filled with joy through encounters with loved ones, connections to strong social networks, and reflections on purposeful lives and powerful memories. As Eric Cassell noted many years ago, the goal of medicine is the relief of suffering. Healing strives for such wholeness and relief, when the words *curing* and *caring* fall short of the mark. A healer strives to cure when possible, moderates suffering when cure is not available, and helps patients transcend suffering when all else fails.

Measured Words

The obligation to carefully choose drug treatments and adjust doses and modes of administration customized to the specific person is hardly a surprising idea to clinicians. There is no one-size-fits-all regimen that suits all patients for all ailments and such a mode of practice would be illogical, given the multiplicity of factors and variables that impinge on such pharmacological choices. The new field of precision medicine postulates that treatments must be selected and adapted based on a fine-grained analysis of genetic and other variations that characterize people and their illnesses. Tumors are deciphered in molecular detail, drug metabolism phenotypes are assessed, T lymphocytes are educated in vitro, and personal behavioral characteristics are evaluated to arrive at a specifically designed recipe for interventions. This emerging discipline recognizes that treatments are increasingly potent but only in highly selected settings, while in other instances there may be limited efficacy yet great toxicity. These careful choices acknowledge the great diversity of people and their ways of living.

Words, metaphors, and those who administer them are equally potent, and sometimes toxic, agents of intervention. Akin to chemical and biological drugs, the power and/or ill effects of words and language are dependent on the precise nature of the recipients, their experiences, attitudes, values, and biological and social characters. There are words that heal and words that harm, and we would do well to conceptualize a pharmacology of words and consider precision metaphors as a branch of precision medicine. Language is as specific as chemical compounds used in therapy and a change of prefix or addition of a comma can alter meaning no less than altering the side chain of a drug. Words can be twisted just as compounds can be rotated sterically with dramatic impact on biological potency in both settings. Words and meanings— and their introduction by a caregiver—are multipotent: using a clock set to advance quickly can convince a diabetic person that time has passed quickly and induce a lower blood sugar than when observing a proper timepiece. There is an interaction among words, drugs, and physicians in that the same dose of active pain medication provides greater relief when presented by a trusted caregiver accompanied by words confident of success. All three—words, drugs, and clinicians—have the power to heal or harm, and each must be administered with proper reflection and due care. In that sense, the triad is the basis for an individualized, customized, relational medicine.

Doctor as Drug

Research on the clinical use of placebos has revealed that the caregiver providing the medication, whether inert or active, is a potent component of the benefits of the treatment. An early articulation of this point is found in a paper entitled "The Doctor Himself as a Therapeutic Agent," read to the American College of Physicians in 1937 by William Houston.[5] The concept of physician as drug was refined by Michael Balint to specify the precise type of doctoring appropriate for the patient in question. These finely tuned subtypes constitute a pharmacology of the personhood of the physician together with the words and gestures being administered. There may be a number of different formulations of the drug, doctor: authoritative guardian, wise mentor, inspirational coach, trusted confidant, objective scientist wedded to the truth, spiritual confessor, affiliated ally, and staunch protector. Each persona is a choice specific to the individual patient at a given point of the illness and must be as carefully selected as a traditional medication or surgical intervention. The trope that caregivers are potent agents immediately suggests that they may also have side effects: indeed, it is a truism in pharmacology that the more potent the drug, the more likely it is to have toxic effects. An authoritative clinician may evoke unwanted feelings of dependence in patients who may wish to take control of their own situations. A patient who is shocked and bewildered at the onset of serious illness will welcome an articulate physician who can provide clear explanations and an offer to accompany and navigate on the joint journey of treatment. One may encounter what can be described as allergic reactions of patients to certain physicians. Previous experiences of unanswered phone calls to a pediatrician by a frantic mother whose child has febrile convulsions may forever sensitize that individual to avoid cold, dispassionate clinicians who are competent, yet fail to offer phone or email support, referring all such inquiries to a local urgent care center. Like many immune allergic responses that are difficult to anticipate, a careful discussion and history may reveal such prior sensitizing experiences. Modeled on careful small exposures of potential allergens, thoughtful probing may uncover points of special vulnerabilities to certain physician-phenotypes and their words.

Stories shared by patients and physicians with first-hand experience of the COVID pandemic reinforce the imperative for a broad understanding of language to encompass all manner of signals shared among the persons involved. Caregivers enrobed in full protective equipment, whose faces cannot be readily seen by patients, choose to wear a large photograph and identifying name tag pinned to the front of their gowns. Conversely, clinicians whose patients are wearing face masks may readily hear the spoken words yet struggle to ascertain the meanings normally signaled by facial expressions such as frowns, grimaces, and smiles. Such unusual circumstances permit us to appreciate the nuanced nature and subtlety of communication, especially in clinical settings. These narratives underline the relational nature of the clinical encounter and the conveyance of meanings through persons and their presence via words, signals, and symbols.

Tailored Relationships

Just as there is no single therapeutic plan to address all illnesses, there is no single mode of clinical encounter suited to all patients. An appreciation of the elements that contribute to the course of the relationship, the persons, words and gestures point to the value of discursive diversity and metaphoric pluralism adapted by a reflective practitioner to achieve the considered goals and objectives developed in concert with the patient. This formulation comes as little surprise to clinicians accustomed to carefully calibrating the administration of cardiac medications adjusted for the patient's weight, serum electrolyte levels, and functional capacities of the kidneys and liver—and, of course, after suitable inquiries regarding known allergies, whether to drugs or to persons. While the process is relational and choices are made with the patient, the responsibility for ensuring that all manner of interventions are the result of reflection and careful consideration rests with the physician. How then does the clinician consider and calibrate words, metaphors, and the self?

Part of the answer flows from the exemplar of pharmacology and the requirement for physicians to be educated in the potency of drugs, their actions, toxicities, and variable dose-response curves that depend on the particular recipient. While medical students absorb a great deal of factual information about pharmaceuticals during their formal studies, it is the experience gained through practice that inculcates the capacity to tailor drugs, doses, and modes of administration to the specificity of each patient. Similarly, the capacity to choose words and stances begins with an awareness of their potency, for both good and ill. The sensitivity to words and language must be accompanied by a learned realization that medicine is a relational encounter between patient and physician that is deeply rooted in the bedrock of language and symbols. Both drugs and words are biopsychosocial in their mode of action that does not recognize a bright line between psyche and soma. While it is relevant (yet rare) to learn of the performative nature of language and metaphors in medical school, the skill to adapt words to the character of the patient grows together with a burgeoning realization through clinical experience of the finely grained diversity and contingent requirements of persons who are ill. Learning that clinical medicine is not a taxonomic ascertainment of diseases but a dyadic process of connection with patients and their specificities, together with a deepening understanding of the entailed imperative for attuned responses, constitutes the maturation of the clinician. At the heart of the clinical enactment is the entanglement of the concerns of the patient manifest as fear, uncertainty, and angst with the careful responses of the physician that provide safety, clarity, and hope.

To use language effectively as part of therapeutic engagement, the physician must understand that the practice of clinical medicine is essentially metaphoric. The language of the dyadic encounter is necessarily figurative—direct, factual speech cannot alone accomplish the goals of the clinician to craft the bond, provide reassurance and guidance, assuage fears, and offer comfort and safe harbor. Scientists develop models of disease expressed in verbal or diagrammatic metaphors, and physicians explain the genesis of illness using concepts of mutated genes, blocked receptors, clogged arteries, and other descriptors from the plumber's craft. Patients depict pain in figurative details (how else can one describe pain?) and their aspirations are often expressed in spiritual tropes. Placebos, like medications, do not simply represent relief—they are the very instruments that can alleviate pain and lift depression. Words in that context are not simply representations of an object in the world, they display performative potency. To choose words wisely and with therapeutic intent, the skilled clinician must appreciate that power.

An awareness of the capacity of words to heal or harm is ideally accompanied by an appreciation of the impact of the clinician as individual and the patient's response to the physician's presence and demeanor. Medical students witness the daily clinical practice of their teachers and are most often inspired and motivated by how their role models attend to and interact with their patients. Students seek to attain the surgical skills or diagnostic acumen of their teachers, but it is the caregivers' attitudes to and respect for their patients that imprint most forcefully on the medical students' nascent clinical identities. Trainees are the first to notice when attending physicians fail to visit their patients and regard them not as persons but as records and images on a computer. Many teachers remain unaware of their influence on their students and have yet to learn of the phenomenon of pedagogical presence as the educational counterpart to clinical presence.

Customized responses to the nuanced concerns that weigh on patients entail a carefully attuned mode of clinical listening. Attending to the symptoms described by a patient in order to arrive at a tentative diagnosis of pneumonia does not entail the same careful listening required to excavate the as-yet unarticulated fear and uncertainty that attends an impending hospital admission for treatment. Perhaps the physician understands the clinical presentation to indicate a simple bronchitis while the patient anticipates a diagnosis of a COVID pneumonia and the prospect of a lengthy quarantine and risks to family members at home. Thus, the concept of tailored and individualized responsiveness to the evolving situation of the patient demands an open, nonjudgmental, albeit analytic, form of listening that probes for subtexts and hidden meanings that patients may find difficult to express and share. The physician bears a duty to ascertain the deeper demands for care that may underlie the initial concerns presented on arrival. Careful attentiveness has the ancillary benefit of signaling respect for the person who seeks care—that the individual is owed a hearing—and demonstrates that the concerns of the patient regarding encounters, mode of discourse, and involvement in decision-making are uppermost in the mind of the physician. These characteristics of engagement provide a permissive context for the careful unfolding of therapeutic words and a reassuring presence.

Humility

The physician's capacity to heal requires a combination of presence and humility—attributes that at first seem antithetical or paradoxical. Presence signals a mastery of the knowledge and skills to meet the demands of accurate interpretations and appropriate interventions and management. Perseverance indicates an engagement with the patient and a commitment to fulfill the mandate of care combined with an awareness that the duties of the clinician must be carried out with honesty and diligence. Presence in the sense of being-there demonstrates a capability and offers a promise to assuage fears and offer safety. Even as presence has a requisite quality of authoritativeness, it also contains a hint of the authoritarian. Thus, the sense of being-there must be self-regulated so that it does not transform into being-in-charge with its risk of an overbearing paternalism. Humility is the attribute that provides a necessary counterpoise to diminish the risk of an intrusive attitude in the demeanor of the clinician.

To be clear, this is not humility as meekness or lowliness and self-abasement. Rather, humility is the attribute of regard for the other in the same or greater measure as regard for the self. It is an esteem that is other-directed rather than solipsistic; a preference for the dyadic connection, not a monadic cocoon. This form of humility searches for and celebrates the good in others rather than in reference to self. The power of this concept, most expressively articulated in Emmanuel Levinas' philosophy of alterity, resides in the fundamental imperative of responding to the call of the Other, whose call emanates directly from suffering and need. In medicine, this refers to the demand of the suffering patient for the care and caring of the physician— a demand expressed not only for the relief of suffering but also for recognition of the patient's humanity, dignity, and worth. Responses to such calls from the suffering patient that provide relief and honor the value of the Other as person are powerful and necessary elements of clinical care. What underscores the radical nature of Levinas' articulation of alterity is that the obligation to respond is unidirectional: "the intersubjective relation is a non symmetrical relation ... I am responsible for the Other without waiting for reciprocity."[6] Finally, alterity connotes that the practice of medicine is grounded in a relationship to the Other that entails trust, confidence, security, and self-worth—all necessary prerequisites for healing.

In the dyadic patient–physician relationship, the clinician's humility entails many pragmatic and significant benefits. Responsibility for the welfare of the patient and respect for the patient's dignity and worth spur the physician to make space for the being and words of the counterpart in the dyad. Such deference is readily evident in addressing persons in an egalitarian interaction and the acceptance that patients may be vulnerable but deserving of esteem should prevent the untimely, if not rude, interruptions of the patient's rendition of the story of illness that have been documented in many studies over at least a half-century. The respectful clinician sits at the bedside or next to the patient in the clinic, again signaling an interaction between equals that also avoids an authoritarian stance from on-high. To avoid confusion, it is worth noting that we speak of equals in deserving dignity and esteem, while clearly differing in vulnerability or relevant skills. Harvey Chochinov introduced the phrase "dignity conserving care"[7] to refer to the need for patients to be regarded with respect by their caregivers. The humble clinician, respectful of the words of the patient, reaps the added incentive to careful listening. After all, if the physician presumes that the patient is right, then it is a matter of good clinical practice to attend to the narrative and its nuances, as it provides clues to the nature of the ailment and hints at pathways to treatment. Creating an uninterrupted window in time also provides an opportunity for the clinician to reflect carefully on the language and demeanor of the person seeking care.[8] The patience motivated by the objective of gleaning details and cryptic elements of the story has the ancillary benefit of averting premature closure, anchoring, and confirmation bias, three well-known pitfalls in clinical diagnosis. The impetus for rapid turnaround and high clinic volumes spur busy and harried physicians to make quick assessments based on sketchy details that increase the probability of medical errors and unnecessary return visits to clinics and emergency rooms. One powerful preventive to avert poor outcomes and high costs is a modicum of humility of a clinician who is able to temper an inflated ego and moderate an overestimation of clinical skills. Modesty is a potent tonic both for the humble physician and the grateful patient.

A mutually respectful dyadic encounter enables a mode of joint reflection, an interchange of ideas and perspectives characteristic of a fruitful collaboration and thus of particular significance in the clinical domain. A clinical story is co-constructed at the outset of the encounter and evolves as a shared production over the course of illness. A consensus of understanding is the desired outcome. En route, disagreements are aired, not buried, and the patient will be comfortable in revealing concerns and choices knowing they will be considered with care and responsiveness. The manifest willingness and ability of the clinician to listen carefully assure the patient of the physician's engagement, competence, patience, and a capacity to acknowledge the patient's uniqueness and humanity. Recognition of individuality and even idiosyncrasy counters the current polarized climate of identity politics and strange taxonomies that categorize persons based on simplistic and misleading labels. The clinical stance of humility manifest as regard for the other avoids classifications of persons and patients whether grounded in diagnostic groupings of diseases or superficial labels of race, age, ethnicity, or gender. Respectful attention to the primacy of the other cannot be as an exemplar of a set and certainly not with respect to a banal notion of diversity. What demands and garners the physician's respect is the individual who is unique in richness and complexity and whose identifiable voice calls for help.

Healing Metaphors

Healing metaphors can be understood in at least two ways. If the word *healing* is read as a verb, then it points to a process of making whole or repairing metaphors that may be broken or ill-considered. If certain metaphors in clinical practice are harmful or noxious, perhaps we should eliminate them from our medical or even societal repertoire. The many unfortunate consequences of military metaphors in medicine and other examples of figurative language that undermine the confidence and self-esteem of the elderly have been noted. Certain tropes remind patients of illnesses they would sooner forget; some women who are well after successful treatment for breast cancer have expressed a desire to survive beyond being survivors and to return to being ordinarily and boringly healthy.

By contrast, *healing* as an adjective reminds us that words relieve fears, diminish shock, lessen confusion, offer comfort and guidance; the words acknowledge as worthy patients who feel isolated and frightened in the midst of chaos and uncertainty. Healing metaphors are those that respond to the patient's existential concerns, expressed or submerged, and that are provided by a physician to whom both patients and words matter. Both uses of the word *healing*, as verb and adjective, indicate that metaphors can harm. To return to the analogy between words and drugs, placebos, whether invoked by the words or the presence of the caregiver, may be accompanied by nocebo effects, that is, untoward or undesirable outcomes, just as potent drugs may bring side effects. A recent study demonstrated that in many instances the side effects that led patients to stop taking a prescribed statin were due to a nocebo effect and were not induced by the active ingredient.[9] Similarly, a physician who presents a strong supportive presence may bring an assurance of accompaniment to most patients while creating mild anxiety to some who may sense an impending loss of freedom to choose alternatives.

A duty to offer care and responsiveness indicates that the imperative to use metaphors that have the potential to heal becomes a matter of awareness and selectivity in language akin to choosing pharmacological and surgical interventions. Painstaking choices will also have the ancillary benefit of diminishing the use of toxic metaphors that can be rendered obsolete and eliminated from common use. One cautionary note: certain metaphors that are not helpful for most patients may yet be helpful for highly selected persons and situations, just as very toxic drugs may be administered in rare instances. Metaphors of battle and war that are deleterious to most patients can find a niche in caring for those persons for whom real and metaphoric fights are a way of being. The imperatives of awareness and selectivity in language can be understood as incumbent on clinicians, institutions of health care, and society writ large. Individual clinicians have a duty of knowing their patients and reflecting on the choices of words and metaphors best suited to their concerns. A patient's sense of chaos and helplessness can be assuaged by information and clear instructions; a fear of abandonment can be met with accompaniment; suffering requires the comfort of presence and a commitment to provide care and stay the course; and the degradation of a hospital robe and a loss of personhood can be tempered by respect and an egalitarian demeanor. Clinicians can learn, through reflection and feedback, to avoid stimuli with nocebo effects. Instructing a patient to summon a caregiver when the pain begins instills an expectation of a painful recovery. It may be helpful to simply state that a caregiver is here should something arise. Telling a patient about high-risk groups can be recast as "You may wish to learn about certain preventive measures." Rather than warning a diabetic patient about foot ulcers, a recommendation for routine podiatric care to maintain healthy feet can achieve the same objective without aversive conditioning. Just as nocebos can be sins of commission, a lost opportunity to provide a placebo is a failure of omission. The leader of a care team in a hospital setting can add to the initial introductory meeting with the patient a supportive comment that "we are members of a health care team and I, together with my colleagues, will be responsible for your care and well-being during your stay in hospital. You or your family can reach me with the contact information that I will leave in the chart." Similarly, an anesthesiologist meeting a patient the night before surgery can end the encounter by noting "you will see me again in the operating room area before you are sedated. I will be with you until the procedure is completed and you are transferred to the recovery room." The promise of accompaniment by a friendly caregiver can moderate preoperative stress and anxiety and permit a restful sleep by a frightened patient. In brief, not providing a word of comfort is tantamount to forgetting to prescribe an indicated medication. The clinical literature is replete with research on the effects of medical errors that have resulted in major efforts on patient safety and reduction of morbidity. Perhaps the taxonomy of medical errors can acknowledge and list linguistic faults of commission and omission as clinical errors so that programs of training will include sensitivity to words and metaphors for their potency and therapeutic effects.

This brings us to the responsibilities of institutions, including hospitals, clinics, long-term care facilities, and other entities engaged in health care services. The adoption of safe practices regarding the placement of central venous infusion lines did not simply follow the publication of research showing a dramatic drop in rates of infection with the use of simple, but stringent, hygienic procedures. Behaviors of hospital-based professionals changed only when the institutions made such safeguards mandatory under pressure from insurance companies that insisted that the costs of such avoidable infections would no longer be covered. There was a quick response and the national rates of infections dropped dramatically. Similarly, individuals must be supported by institutional policies that reflect awareness of the influence of language on outcomes and, therefore, costs. Such policies could include the avoidance of the word *negative* when reporting the results of blood tests and other investigations that yield normal findings. Patients attuned to words and whose awareness may be impaired by illness readily misconstrue the word *negative* to mean a bad outcome. After all, in the non-clinical world, a negative bank balance and a negative reply to an offer to purchase are not happy outcomes. Forms to request consent for procedures should be truthful in describing potential side effects; yet, there are many ways to frame the possibilities. Rather than simply stating that the placement of a central venous line (portacath) can lead to serious blood infections, the information might be restated as, "Our caregivers complete a careful skin cleansing and wear gloves and masks to prevent infections that have been known to occur. Do not hesitate to ask us if you have any questions." Institutional policy can support a decision by the anesthesia department to provide headsets with comforting words and music for patients undergoing anesthesia for surgical procedures. The impact of this modest intervention was demonstrated in an empirical randomized multicenter trial, in which patients under anesthesia who listened to audios of music and positive therapeutic suggestions experienced less postoperative pain and required smaller opioid doses after surgery than patients in the control arm who received blank tapes.[10] Similar simple nonpharmacological interventions require a thoughtful institutional culture. Leaders can provide training to those responsible for moving patients from their rooms to other parts of the hospital to introduce themselves to patients and offer assurance that they will accompany them to the relevant imaging unit and will be responsible for their safe and timely return to their rooms. Too many patients are left undraped on a gurney in a hallway, feeling abandoned in a strange department of a large impersonal institution.

Daily small decisions by individuals to use carefully selected words that heal and support by thoughtful institutional policies provide models and exemplars for dissemination. While it may be helpful to support a patient by noting that postoperative pain is common, it is important to immediately add that such after-effects can and will be treated promptly. However, it does not help to tell such a person that "you may feel like you were hit by a truck." Both types of comments may become self-fulfilling prophecies—the latter may lead to increased pain and fear, the former to the comfort that relief will be readily available. The cumulative and incremental effects of many small actions enable cultural change that proceeds slowly until an inflection point is reached, and a process of acceleration is launched. Intentional campaigns to alter behaviors can promote and enhance the use of salutary metaphors, though the elimination of those that are noxious may require longer-term changes in linguistic habits. Nonetheless, the burgeoning use of metaphors that heal can displace those that require healing. There are many examples of sweeping changes in the use of words, once commonly accepted and now understood as pejorative and demeaning. Happily, we no longer speak of crippled children, we appreciate that eugenics was about more than happy families, and have discarded the discriminatory labels once used to classify persons with intellectual disabilities. All these words are now gone from our daily lexicons yet were in common use in civil society prior to World War II—less than a century ago. These changes demonstrate the power of social norms in altering how we describe and see the world. Moreover, linguistic usage is likely to evolve ever more quickly under the influence of social media and global networks that traffic rapidly in words and ideas.

Physicians and Language

The key to engaged relationships enacted in healing language is the recognition that both patients and words come in almost infinite varieties and selecting the metaphors best suited for the individual patient seeking care is a primary clinical duty. Clinical medicine depends on the physician's adaptability to the particular through a process of listening, reflection, and calibration of words. The underlying skill is a hermeneutic attention gained through cumulative clinical experience and directed to three sets of living texts: the patient, the narrative, and the self. In all instances, the object and medium of analysis is language. The narrative of the patient is expressed in words that require interpretation to be usefully apprehended and the interactive nature of learning the story of illness is itself an analytic process. Subtexts, hidden meanings, implicit fears and concerns must be unearthed and deciphered.

The patient is also a text whose demeanor, behavior, and physiognomy are symbolic and rife with meaning. The patient is a product of time and experiences that shape character, emotions, and responses to illness—these are not immediately evident in the direct story of falling ill but can be relevant to understanding the genesis of the signs and symptoms. Thus, both the patient's narrative and lived experiences are texts of interest to the clinician. The third element that requires interpretation is the physician who must develop an awareness of the impact of the doctor's presence and words on the well-being of the patient. This reflective skill is more complex and demands a self-critical gaze that is not readily acquired. With cumulative clinical experiences that are assessed forthrightly and perhaps with the benefit of discussions with trusted colleagues, physicians can acquire the craftsman's skills necessary to the clinical mandate.

The emphasis on language, words, and metaphors as an integral part of physician-ship points to the relevance of the humanities as sources for clinical work. Clinical medicine requires a curiosity and regard for people, a sensitivity to and an understanding of language and how it works, and an appreciation of human relationships. Humanities in this sense refers to a study of humans, their histories and narratives. It does not connote the humane, that is, of kindness and other moral virtues, but the relevance of the human disciplines (*Geisteswissenschaften*) to medical education. Medicine, comprising the duties and practices of the physician, entails a knowledge of people, an interest in how they live, a desire to understand how they speak, a mandate to know how they fall ill, and a commitment to support their recoveries—all these, coupled with the pragmatic skills of engagement and hermeneutics.

Clinical medicine requires an array of skills, understood as craftmanship deployed by a prudent physician capable of wise judgment. Craftmanship demands practiced skills that become second nature with time and repetition and prudent choices are grounded in cumulative clinical experiences and the subsequent recursive reflections on outcomes. The virtue of prudence of the careful, wise clinician, alloyed with the pragmatic skills of the craftsman and tempered by the moral virtue of humility, constitute a faithful rendering of the physician as person and as healer. Our continuing commitment to train young physicians to share those aspirations and to serve our patients clinically in congruence with that vision will enable us to fulfill the vocation of physicianship.

Afterword

The limits of my language means the limits of my world.
—Ludwig Wittgenstein

This book is a co-constructed narrative, shaped by the many scholars whose works provided pathways and insights and sources of inspiration, and inflected by discussions and collaborations with colleagues and students whom I have had the good fortune to encounter on my journey. This extended essay shares thoughts and ideas, my own and those of others, that demonstrate the power of words and language in the enactment of medicine in the clinical relationship between patient and physician. The book is neither a pedagogical primer on correct usage nor is it an exhaustive analysis of metaphors that should be used and others which must necessarily be shunned. Rather, my aim is, in the first instance, to stimulate a reflective awareness among clinicians and their current and future patients—that is, all of us—of the importance and impact of language at the very heart of medical care. I have learned from class discussions with medical students that while their newly minted stories of interactions with patients reveal an authentic enthusiasm for clinical work, they are unaware of the imperative of listening and of the bilateral effects of words. In part, this is due to the rather rigid formats of the standardized clinical interview and case report that are promulgated in medical curricula. Medical students and residents are often too busy filling in the slots and checking the boxes of the electronic health record to pay attention to the patient, who is, after all, the source of the story. Nonetheless, when students are prompted to reflect on their narratives and those of their classmates, they readily appreciate and begin to heed the nuances of words and body language in their clinical duties.

Second, sensitivity to language immediately entails an attentiveness to patients and a realization that clinical work may be bolstered by laboratory data and imaging results, but it necessitates engagement with the patient if it is to succeed in its mission of care. To be clear, the intent is not to call for a return to a rosy yesteryear of the "good old days" that were wonderful only in retrospect through sepia-toned lenses. Medical care must inevitably attend to persons whether the immediate aim is to cure, care, or console. In brief, physicians must become enchanted by those persons who are patients, rather than bewitched by the marvels of science.

Words and expressions change with mindsets that are responsive to societal shifts of values—there are many phrases once thought to be acceptable within social norms that are now considered pejorative and beyond the pale. What remains foundational in clinical practice is the demand for an adaptive, flexible, thoughtful, and customized stance of the physician to the patient whose care is the responsibility of the provider. To remain grounded in that reality and to maintain the relational when it is under threat demands a steadfast commitment by individual clinicians to the duty of care.

My own awareness of the realities and foibles of language in the clinic was spurred by a paper published in 1986 by William Donnelly with the intriguing title, "Medical Language as Symptom: Doctor Talk in Teaching Hospitals," which was a wonderful exploration of the vernacular. A search for additional sources on language and clinical work led to a two-volume treatise by Eric Cassell, titled *Talking with Patients*, based on many hours of audiotapes of actual clinical interviews. This work remains an underutilized resource for medical education and medical linguistics more generally, as it attends not only to words but to prosody, pronoun choices, and other audible clues to the clinical interaction. An interest in English as language, seemingly common among those whose first language is other than English, led to a small volume by George Lakoff and Mark Johnson, *Metaphors We Live By*, which opened the door not simply to words in the clinic but rather to the metaphors that populate the discourse of medicine, both among professionals and among English speakers more generally.

The importance of stories in clinical work was highlighted by an elective seminar for senior medical students on the language of medicine and informal meetings with medical students throughout their clinical training. The trainees expressed an eagerness to share stories about their patients and their own experiences as nascent physicians. These students' stories made clear that medical curricula did not offer such opportunities and clinical training paid little attention to this feature of caring for patients. Rita Charon developed the important theme of narrative medicine and I had the good fortune of learning from her during her visits to McGill University and my own visit to her group at Columbia University. These encounters extended the interfaces between medicine, words, and metaphors from an interesting phenomenon of clinical work to a deeper appreciation of the crucial importance of language in the clinical encounter and its participants.

An encounter with a McGill medical alumnus, David Holbrooke, led to the next stage of the project on language and medicine with the participation of Megan O'Connor as a postdoctoral fellow. O'Connor, who had completed her doctoral work at Oxford, used her research skills to prepare an annotated bibliography of historical sources of military metaphors in medical and classical writings. This material was then expanded by Nora Hutchinson, a medical student pursuing a research initiative with the support of a McGill student research bursary. She enriched the array of important archival materials and prepared a survey of the appearances of war metaphors in two international medical journals. A second medical student, Douglas

Slobod, examined English corpora for instances of the military tropes and authored a paper entitled "Military Metaphors and Friendly Fire."

A sabbatical leave in 2007–2008 supported by the Arnold and Blema Steinberg Foundation offered a year of seminars, readings, and meetings with colleagues at Harvard's Department of Social Medicine and at Boston University's Department of Philosophy. I benefited from encounters with Allan Brandt, Arthur Kleinman, the late Leon Eisenberg and the seminar series on medical anthropology hosted by Byron and Mary-Jo Good. Alfred Tauber was a thoughtful host and guide at Boston University, where I learned a great deal from an informal reading group on Heidegger and Dewey led by Victor Kestenbaum, with participation by Al and Maria Miller.

On my return to McGill at the end of the sabbatical, I benefitted from an academic home in close proximity to the members of the Department of Social Studies of Medicine and the seminars and discussions dedicated to the application of the social sciences and history to the study of medicine. Judy Segal, a visiting professor to that department, offered an opportunity to learn about the rhetorical viewpoint and shared her insights on the humanities in medical education. An important and most enjoyable project that brought together many strands in the teaching of medical students was a collaborative adventure with Eric Cassell and Donald Boudreau as co-authors of a proposal for the design of a medical curriculum that appeared in book form in 2018 as *Physicianship and the Rebirth of Medical Education*. A project led by another visitor to McGill, Edvin Schei, involved Donald Boudreau and myself in an analysis of reflection in medical care and education that culminated in a paper entitled "Reflection in Medical Education: Intellectual Humility, Discovery, and Know-How."

Chapter 11 on the physician–patient relationship draws on the work carried out by Michael Saraga that began with his stay as a visiting professor at McGill and thereafter in a collaboration with Donald Boudreau and me. This wonderful collegial working group of friends continues (an academic entertainment) and has been for me a wonderful source of ideas and reflections, many of which are noted in this chapter and more deeply developed in the cited publications by Saraga et al.

The particular and unique contributions to this volume by several individuals warrant special mention. Victor Kestenbaum read the initial chapters of the book in early draft form. Megan O'Connor, Nora Hutchinson, and Rose-Anna Foley offered helpful comments on individual chapters. Donald Boudreau patiently read the entire manuscript, and provided thoughtful input and feedback. I am grateful for his long-standing collaboration, collegiality, and friendship. Sylvia Fuks Fried offered unflagging support and guidance throughout the preparation of this volume. Her recommendations on organization and structure, and gracious critiques of tone and style are gratefully appreciated. I extend my thanks to Andrea Knobloch and her editorial colleagues at Oxford University Press for their fine work and expertise.

Sacvan Bercovitch was my guiding spirit to the treasures of the Widener Library during my sabbatical year in Boston and a mentor whose wisdom and deep learning infused our discussions over afternoon tea. Saki's belief in the value of the work inspired the research and the project. I miss our meetings, his gentle collegiality, and his friendship. I dedicate this book to Saki's memory.

Notes

Chapter 1

1. Grondin, p. 100.
2. Richardson, p. 282.
3. Taylor, p. 23, fn. 31.
4. Oxford English Dictionary Online, empathy, definition 2. https://www.oed.com/view/Entry/61284#eid5524311
5. Grondin, p. 117.

Chapter 2

1. Williams et al.
2. Heritage et al.
3. Phillips & Hickner (2005).
4. Pellegrini et al.
5. Romer, p. 197.
6. Romer, p. 194.
7. Boroditzsky.
8. Woolf, p. 16.
9. Sontag, p. 4.
10. Fuks (2018).
11. Hacking (2007).
12. Mullan.
13. Hacking (1995).
14. Deber.
15. Segal (2019), p. 172.

Chapter 3

1. Lakoff & Johnson, p. 455.
2. Fowler & Fowler, p. 116.
3. Fowler & Fowler, p. 116.
4. Deignan, p. 255.
5. Boers, p. 50.
6. Pollio et al., p. 143.
7. Sontag, p. 3.
8. Snævarr, p. 75.
9. Snævarr, p. 112.
10. Cohn (1987a), p. 692.
11. Cohn (1987a), p. 690.

12. Cohn (2001), p. 107.
13. Cohn (1987a), p. 704.
14. Cohn (1987a), p. 708.
15. Cohn (2001), p. 113.
16. Cohn (1987b), p. 24.
17. Cohn (2001), p. 101.
18. Cohn (2001), p. 114.
19. Cohn (2001), p. 108.
20. Cohn (2001), p. 113.
21. Cohn (1987a), p. 716.
22. Cameron & Low, p. 82.

Chapter 4

1. American Cancer Society, Our history. https://www.cancer.org/about-us/who-we-are/our-history.html
2. Women's Field Army poster. https://www.gfwc.org/exhibits-microsite/vex1/images/6E703067-3230-40FA-BEA2-963474583617.jpg
3. *BMJ* editorial, 1934;1:1127. https://doi.org/10.1136/bmj.1.3833.1127
4. Lerner, p. 74.
5. Lerner, p. 74.
6. Lerner, p. 77.
7. de Kruif.
8. CDC, CDC organization. https://www.cdc.gov/about/organization/cio.htm
9. Hoffman.
10. Hoffman.
11. Sontag, p. 7.
12. Sontag, p. 9.
13. Sontag, p. 17.
14. Bernstein.
15. Demmen et al.
16. Demmen et al., p. 218.
17. Demmen et al., p. 220.
18. Demmen et al., p. 220.

Chapter 5

1. A comprehensive treatment of the many sources of these metaphors will require a more finely grained historical analysis than can be achieved in this single chapter whose aim is to point to the different strands that contributed to the contemporary idiom.
2. Sontag, p. 66.
3. Sontag, p. 66.
4. Montgomery, p. 139.
5. Montgomery, p. 151.
6. Cited in Rather (1982), pp. 143–144; Schultz-Schultzenstein.
7. Virchow (1847), cited in Rather (1982), p. 145.

8. Virchow (1885).

9. Rather (1982), p. 145.

10. Virchow (1847), cited in Otis, p. 22.

11. Osler, cited by Cushing, p. 1101.

12. Zinsser, p. 14.

13. Editorial (1860, April 7). The health of the city. *New York Times*, 4. https://timesmachine. nytimes.com/timesmachine/1860/04/07/76649693.html?pageNumber=4

14. Editorial (1861, June 17). Military hygiene. *New York Times*, 4. https://timesmachine. nytimes.com/timesmachine/1861/06/17/355615412.html?pageNumber=4

15. Letter to the Editor (March 24, 1864). *New York Times*.

16. To Correspondents (1848, February, 27). The war against disease and death. *Lloyd's Weekly London Newspaper*, 6. https://www.britishnewspaperarchive.co.uk/viewer/bl/0000078/ 18480227/014/0006

17. Wednesday's Post Continued (1848, July, 17). Purifying bed feathers. *Aris's Birmingham Gazette*, 4. https://www.britishnewspaperarchive.co.uk/viewer/bl/0000196/18480717/ 009/0004

18. von Helmont, cited by Pagel, p. 420.

19. Paracelsus, p. 443.

20. Sydenham et al., pp. 38–39.

21. Sydenham et al., p. 115.

22. Boerhaave (1740), p. 12.

23. Brissot, cited in Rather & Frerichs, p. 188.

24. Campanella, cited in Rather & Frerichs, p. 202.

25. Campanella citing Galen, cited in Rather & Frerichs, p. 203.

26. Niebyl, p. 155.

27. Campanella, cited in Rather & Frerichs, p. 202.

28. Paracelsus, p. 429.

29. Paracelsus, p. 443.

30. Paracelsus, cited in Pagel, p. 449.

31. von Helmont, cited in Pagel, p. 420.

32. von Helmont, cited in Pagel, p. 442.

33. Sydenham et al., p. 60.

34. Boerhaave (1715), p. 115.

35. Bacon, p. 160.

36. OED, *canker*, defn 4a.

37. OED, *cancer*, defn 3b.

38. Grünpeck, cited in Moore & Solomon, p. 7.

39. Grünpeck, cited in Moore & Solomon, p. 11.

40. Donne, p. 351.

41. Perkins et al., p. 501, cited in Wear, p. 7.

42. Perkins et al., p. 153, cited in Wear, p. 9.

43. Perkins et al, p. 365, cited in Wear, p. 14.

44. Perkins et al., p. 794.

45. Nutton, p. 47.

46. Nutton, p. 47.

47. Nutton, p. 47.

48. Nutton, p. 48.
49. Jacobs.
50. Fletcher, p. 201.
51. Fletcher, p. 203.
52. Temkin, p. 457.
53. Douglas, p. 2.
54. Douglas, p. 48.
55. Douglas, p. 9.
56. Becker, p. 49.
57. Becker, p. 47.
58. Becker, p. 47.
59. Becker, p. 87.
60. Becker, p. 63.

Chapter 6

1. Fissell, p. 94.
2. Mutter, p. 3.
3. Mutter, p. 6.
4. Rosenberg (2002), p. 240.
5. Baziak & Dentan, p. 263.
6. Fissell, p. 96.
7. Fissell, p. 103.
8. Jewson (1976), p. 228.
9. Jewson (1976), p. 225.
10. Jewson (1976), p. 237.
11. Zhong and Liljenquist, p. 1451.
12. Kalanthroff et al., p. 6.
13. Rosenberg (1987), p. 216.
14. Hu, p. 1.
15. Rawcliffe, p. 19.
16. Hudson & Morton, p. 1495.
17. Frascatoro.
18. Qin et al.
19. O'Shea et al.
20. Ross, p. 40, re: AIDS.
21. Ross, p. 44.
22. Ross, p. 55.
23. Latour, p. 8.
24. Tomes, p. 52.
25. Tomes, p. 62.
26. Tomes, p. 10.
27. Tomes, p. 135.
28. Tomes, p. 11.
29. Tomes, p. 48.
30. Tomes, p. 48.

31. Tomes, p. 186.
32. Tomes, p. 203.
33. Tomes, p. 125.
34. Tomes, p. 124.
35. King.
36. Hauser & Schwarz (2015), p. 68.
37. Hauser & Schwarz (2020).
38. Tauber (2016).
39. OED, *minister* (n), defn. 5.
40. OED, *minister* (v), defn. 8.

Chapter 7

1. Ryan & Ryan.
2. Hawkins (1984), p. 234.
3. Ryan & Ryan, p. 19.
4. Ryan & Ryan, p. 102.
5. Ryan & Ryan, p. 410.
6. Ryan & Ryan, p. 215.
7. Hawkins (1984), p. 241.
8. Hawkins (1984), p. 241.
9. Ryan & Ryan, p. 212.
10. Ryan & Ryan, p. 241.
11. Ryan & Ryan, p. 231.
12. Ryan & Ryan, p. 314.
13. Ryan & Ryan, p. 332.
14. Ryan & Ryan, p. 102.
15. Ryan & Ryan, p. 53.
16. Ryan & Ryan, p. 177.
17. Ryan & Ryan, p. 194.
18. Ryan & Ryan, p. 374.
19. Hawkins (1999), p. 30.
20. Hawkins (1984), p. 239.
21. Ryan & Ryan, p. 197.
22. Ryan & Ryan, p. 307.
23. Ryan & Ryan, p. 354.
24. Ryan & Ryan, p. 390.
25. Ryan & Ryan, p. 376.
26. Ryan & Ryan, p. 395.
27. Hawkins (1999), p. 21.
28. Hawkins (1999), p. 21.
29. Ryan & Ryan, p. 359.
30. Ryan & Ryan, p. 390.
31. Hawkins (1999), p. 68.
32. Hawkins (1999), p. 68.
33. Hawkins (1999), p. 68.

34. Hawkins (1984), p. 246.
35. Hawkins (1999), p. 73.
36. Hawkins (1999), p. 73.
37. Reisfield & Wilson, p. 4024.
38. May, p. 21.
39. May, p. 66.
40. Hawkins (1990).
41. Hawkins (1999), p. 76.

Chapter 8

1. Harper.
2. Harper.
3. George et al. (2016), p. 23.
4. George (2010), p. 587.
5. George (2010), p. 587.
6. George (2010), p. 587.
7. George & Whitehouse (2014), p. 127.
8. Qiu et al., p. 689.
9. George (2010), p. 587.
10. George & Whitehouse (2014), p. 120.
11. Stibbe, p. 182.
12. Nie et al., p. 8.
13. Nie et al., p. 8.
14. Nie et al., p. 9.
15. Nie et al., pp. 9–10.
16. Annas, p. 747.
17. Annas, p. 746.
18. Canguilhem, p. 40.
19. Canguilhem, p. 88.
20. Canguilhem, p. 228.
21. Canguilhem, p. 91.
22. Hawkins (1999), p. 82.
23. Hawkins (1999), p. 83.
24. Hawkins (1999), p. 86.
25. Woolf, p. 34.
26. Reisfield & Wilson, p. 4026.
27. Reisfield & Wilson, p. 4026.
28. Nie et al., p. 10.
29. Nie et al., p. 11.
30. Reisfield & Wilson, p. 4026.
31. Semino et al., p. 63.
32. Perrault & O'Keefe, p. 14.
33. Perrault & O'Keefe, p. 14.
34. Perrault & O'Keefe, p. 14.
35. Hawkins (1999), p. 83.

36. Reisfield & Wilson, p. 4026.
37. Penson et al., p. 710.
38. Penson et al., p. 711.
39. Broyard, p. 50.
40. Frank, p. 203.
41. Frank, p. 204.
42. Frank, p. 205.
43. Frank, p. 204.
44. Frank, p. 205.
45. Frank, p. 205.
46. Reisfield & Wilson, p. 4026.
47. Perrault & O'Keefe, p. 14.

Chapter 9

1. Ospina et al.
2. Boudreau et al.
3. Jagosh et al.
4. Park et al. (1992).
5. Jackson, p. 1624.
6. Fiumara.
7. Fiumara, p. 111.
8. Fiumara, p. 145.
9. Fiumara, p. 144.
10. Frank, p. 198.
11. Frank, p. 199.
12. Frank, p. 200.
13. Frank, p. 210.
14. Spiro, p. 1177.
15. Smith, pp. xv–xvi.
16. Scott et al., p. 319.
17. Levenstein et al., p. 24.
18. Vico, cited in Fiumara, p. 161; Diamond, p. 25.
19. Fiumara, p. 153.
20. Fiumara, p. 57.
21. Fiumara, p. 28.
22. Fiumara, p. 85.

Chapter 10

1. Haygarth, p. 16.
2. Quincy, p. 394.
3. De Craen et al., p. 511.
4. Kisner.
5. OED, *placebo*, defn. 4.
6. Thomas.

7. Kaptchuk et al. (2008).
8. Howe et al.
9. Brien et al.
10. Amanzio et al. (2001).
11. Benedetti et al. (2003).
12. Levine & Gordon.
13. Benedetti et al. (2011); Colloca et al. (2004).
14. Park & Covi (1965).
15. Hoenemeyer et al.
16. Benedetti et al. (1999), p. 3647.
17. De la Fuente-Fernandez & Stoessl (2002); De la Fuente-Fernandez et al. (2006).
18. Amanzio & Benedetti (1999).
19. Geuter et al.
20. Mackenzie.
21. Bruner et al.
22. Kamenica et al.
23. Kaptchuk (2011), p. 1849.
24. Kaptchuk (2011), p. 1853.
25. Kaptchuk (2011), p. 1850.
26. Phillips et al. (2001).
27. Gould.
28. Moerman (2013).
29. Kleinman & Becker.
30. Moerman (2002), p. 80.
31. Miller & Colloca, p. 512.
32. Simpson et al.
33. Johnson et al., p. 183.
34. Benedetti (2002), p. 381.
35. Findlay.
36. Miller et al. (2009), p. 519.
37. Kaptchuk (2018), p. 324.
38. Gracely et al.
39. Chen et al.
40. Chen et al., p. 1301.

Chapter 11

1. Flexner.
2. Mishler.
3. Engel (1977), p. 132.
4. Engel (1997).
5. Saraga et al. (2014).
6. Saraga et al. (2014), p. 484.
7. Saraga et al. (2014), p. 491.

8. Johnson et al., p. 183: Balint, p. 249.

9. Mol, p. 74.

10. Mol, p. 84.

11. Mol, p. 62.

12. Mol, p. xi.

13. Salmon & Young (2017), p. 260.

14. Salmon & Hall (2004).

15. Salmon & Hall (2003).

16. Balint, p. 76; Johnson et al., p. 186.

17. Scott et al.

18. Mol, p. 84.

19. Zulman et al., p. 70.

20. Brown-Johnson et al., p. 4.

21. Brown-Johnson et al., p. 4.

22. Stiefel & Bourquin, p. 4.

23. Stiefel & Bourquin, p. 4.

24. Saraga et al. (2014) pp. 487–488.

25. Saraga et al. (2014) pp. 487–488

26. Saraga et al. (2014), p. 491.

27. Saraga et al. (2019b).

28. Saraga et al. (2019a).

29. Saraga et al. (2019b), p. 47.

30. Saraga et al. (2019b), p. 44.

31. Saraga et al. (2019b), p. 44.

32. Saraga et al. (2019b), p. 45.

33. Suchman & Matthews.

34. Saraga et al. (2019b), p. 46.

35. Saraga et al. (2019b), p. 46.

36. Saraga et al. (2019a), p. 1.

37. Saraga et al. (2019a), p. 3.

38. Saraga et al. (2019a), p. 4.

39. Saraga et al. (2019a), p. 4.

40. Saraga et al. (2019a), p. 4.

41. Saraga et al. (2019a), p. 5.

42. Saraga et al. (2019a), p. 6.

43. Saraga et al. (2019a), p. 6.

44. Saraga et al. (2019a), p. 9.

Chapter 12

1. Broyard, p. 11.

2. Ishikawa et al., p. 150.

3. OED, *healing*, n1, defn. 2.

4. OED, *physician*, n, defn 2.

5. Houston.

6. Fuks et al. (2012), p. 119.

7. Chochinov, p. 184.

8. Schei et al.

9. Herrett et al.

10. Nowak et al.

Bibliography

Amanzio, M., & Benedetti, F. (1999). Neuropharmacological dissection of placebo analgesia: Expectation-activated opioid systems versus conditioning-activated specific subsystems. *Journal of Neuroscience, 19*(1), 484–494.

Amanzio, M., Pollo, A., Maggi, G., & Benedetti, F. (2001). Response variability to analgesics: A role for non-specific activation of endogenous opioids. *Pain, 90*(3), 205–215.

Annas, G. J. (1995). Reframing the debate on health care reform by replacing our metaphors. *New England Journal of Medicine, 332*(11), 745–748. https://doi.org/10.1056/NEJM199503163321112

Bacon, F. (1906). *Essays.* JM Dent.

Balint, M. (1972). *The doctor, his patient and the illness* (Rev.). International Universities Press.

Baziak, A. T., & Dentan, R. K. (1960). The language of the hospital and its effects on the patient. *ETC: A Review of General Semantics, 17*(3), 261–268.

Becker, C. L. (2003). *The heavenly city of the eighteenth-century philosophers* (2nd ed.). Yale University Press.

Benedetti, F. (2002). How the doctor's words affect the patient's brain. *Evaluation & the Health Professions, 25*(4), 369–386.

Benedetti, F., Arduino, C., & Amanzio, M. (1999). Somatotopic activation of opioid systems by target-directed expectations of analgesia. *Journal of Neuroscience, 19*(9), 3639–3648.

Benedetti, F., Carlino, E., & Pollo, A. (2011). Hidden administration of drugs. *Clinical Pharmacology and Therapeutics, 90*(5), 651–661. https://doi:10.1038/clpt.2011.206

Benedetti, F., Maggi, G., Lopiano, L., Lanotte, M., Rainero, I., Vighetti, S., & Pollo, A. (2003). Open versus hidden medical treatments: The patient's knowledge about a therapy affects the therapy outcome. *Prevention & Treatment, 6*(1). https://doi.org/10.1037/1522-3736.6.1.61a

Bernstein, C. (2018, May 7). Take control of your health care (exert your patient autonomy). *Harvard Health Letter.* https://www.health.harvard.edu/blog/take-control-of-your-health-care-exert-your-patient-autonomy-2018050713784

Boerhaave, H. (1715). *Boerhaave's aphorisms: Concerning the knowledge and cure of diseases.* Translated from the last edition printed in Latin at Leyden, 1715. With useful observations and explanations, by J. Delacoste, M.D.

Boerhaave, H. (1740). *A treatise on the powers of medicines* (J. Martyn, Trans.). Printed by C. Jephson for John Wilcox.

Boers, F. (1999). When a bodily source domain becomes prominent. In R. W. Gibbs & G. Steen (Eds.), *Metaphor in cognitive linguistics: Selected papers from the Fifth International Cognitive Linguistics Conference, Amsterdam, July 1997* (pp. 47–56). J. Benjamins. https://doi.org/10.1075/cilt.175.04boe

Boroditsky, L. (2012). How the languages we speak shape the ways we think: The FAQs. In M. J. Spivey, M. Joanisse, & K. McRae (Eds.), *The Cambridge handbook of psycholinguistics* (pp. 615–632). Cambridge University Press. https://doi.org/10.1017/CBO9781139029377.042

Boudreau, J. D., Jagosh, J., Slee, R., Macdonald, M. E., & Steinert, Y. (2008). Patients' perspectives on physicians' roles: Implications for curricular reform. *Academic Medicine, 83*(8), 744–753.

Brien, S., Lachance, L., Prescott, P., McDermott, C., & Lewith, G. (2011). Homeopathy has clinical benefits in rheumatoid arthritis patients that are attributable to the consultation process but not the homeopathic remedy: A randomized controlled clinical trial. *Rheumatology, 50*(6), 1070–1082.

Brown-Johnson, C., Schwartz, R., Maitra, A., Haverfield, M. C., Tierney, A., Shaw, J. G., Zionts, D. L., Safaeinili, N., Thadaney Israni, S., Verghese, A., & Zulman, D. M. (2019). What is clinician presence? A qualitative interview study comparing physician and non-physician insights about practices of human connection. *BMJ Open, 9*(11), e030831. https://doi.org/10.1136/bmjopen-2019-030831

Broyard, A. (1998). Doctor, talk to me. *Minnesota Medicine, 81*(2), 8–11.

Bruner, J. S., Postman, L., & Rodrigues, J. (1951). Expectation and the perception of color. *American Journal of Psychology, 64*(2), 216–227.

Cameron, L., & Low, G. (1999). Metaphor. *Language Teaching, 32*(2), 77–96. https://doi.org/10.1017/S0261444800013781

Canguilhem, G. (1991). *The normal and the pathological.* (C. Fawcett, Trans.). Zone Books.

Chen, P.-H. A., Cheong, J. H., Jolly, E., Elhence, H., Wager, T. D., & Chang, L. J. (2019). Socially transmitted placebo effects. *Nature Human Behaviour, 3*, 1295–1305. https://doi.org/10.1038/s41562-019-0749-5

Chochinov, H. M. (2007). Dignity and the essence of medicine: The A, B, C, and D of dignity conserving care. *BMJ, 335*(7612), 184–187.

Cohn, C. (1987a). Sex and death in the rational world of defense intellectuals. *Signs, 12*(4), 687–718.

Cohn, C. (1987b). Slick'ems, glick'ems, Christmas trees, and cookie cutters: Nuclear language and how we learned to pat the bomb. *Bulletin of the Atomic Scientists, 43*(5), 17–24.

Cohn, C. (2001). Sex and death in the rational world of defense intellectuals. In M. Wyer, M. Barbercheck, D. Cookmeyer, H. Ö. Öztürk, & M. L. Wayne (Eds.), *Women, science, and technology* (pp. 101–117). Routledge.

Colloca, L., Lopiano, L., Lanotte, M., & Benedetti, F. (2004). Overt versus covert treatment for pain, anxiety, and Parkinson's disease. *The Lancet Neurology, 3*(11), 679–684.

Cushing, H. (1925). *The life of Sir William Osler.* Clarendon Press.

Deber, R. B., Kraetschmer, N., Urowitz, S., & Sharpe, N. (2005). Patient, consumer, client, or customer: What do people want to be called? *Health Expectations, 8*(4), 345–351.

De Craen, A. J., Kaptchuk, T. J., Tijssen, J. G., & Kleijnen, J. (1999). Placebos and placebo effects in medicine: Historical overview. *Journal of the Royal Society of Medicine, 92*(10), 511–515.

Deignan, A. (2003). Metaphorical expressions and culture: An indirect link. *Metaphor and Symbol, 18*(4), 255–271. https://doi.org/10.1207/S15327868MS1804_3

de Kruif, P. (1930). *Microbe hunters.* Blue Ribbon Books.

De la Fuente-Fernández, R., Lidstone, S., & Stoessl, A. J. (2006). Placebo effect and dopamine release. In P. Riederer, H. Reichmann, M. B. Youdim, & M. Gerlach (Eds.), *Parkinson's disease and related disorders* (pp. 415–418). Springer.

De la Fuente-Fernandez, R., & Stoessl, A. J. (2002). The placebo effect in Parkinson's disease. *Trends in Neurosciences, 25*(6), 302–306.

Demmen, J., Semino, E., Demjén, Z., Koller, V., Hardie, A., Rayson, P., & Payne, S. (2015). A computer-assisted study of the use of violence metaphors for cancer and end of life by patients, family carers and health professionals. *International Journal of Corpus Linguistics, 20*(2), 205–231.

Diamond, S. (1977). On reading Vico. *Dialectical Anthropology, 2*(1–4), 19.

Donne, J. (1990). *John Donne* (J. Carey, Ed.). Oxford University Press.

Donnelly, W. J. (1986). Medical language as symptom: Doctor talk in teaching hospitals. *Perspectives in Biology and Medicine, 30*(1), 81–94.

Douglas, M. (2002). *Purity and danger: An analysis of concept of pollution and taboo.* Routledge.

Engel, G. L. (1977). The need for a new medical model: A challenge for biomedicine. *Science, 196*(4286), 129–136.

Engel, G. L. (1997). From biomedical to biopsychosocial: Being scientific in the human domain. *Psychosomatics*, *38*(6), 521–528. https://doi.org/http://dx.doi.org/10.1016/S0033-3182(97)71396-3

Findley, T. (1953). The placebo and the physician. *Medical Clinics of North America*, *37*(6), 1821–1826.

Fissell, M. E. (1991). The disappearance of the patient's narrative and the invention of hospital medicine. In R. French & A. Wear (Eds.), *British medicine in an age of reform* (pp. 92–109). Routledge.

Fiumara, G. C. (1990). *The other side of language: A philosophy of listening.* Routledge.

Fletcher, A. (2012). *Allegory: The theory of a symbolic mode.* Princeton University Press.

Flexner, A. (1910). Medical Education in the United States and Canada Bulletin Number Four (The Flexner Report). The Carnegie Foundation for the Advancement of Teaching.

Fowler, H. W., & Fowler, F. G. (1908). *The King's English abridged for school use.* Clarendon Press.

Fracastoro, G. (1720). *Syphilis sive morbus gallicus.* Lud. Cyaneus.

Frank, A. W. (1998). Just listening: Narrative and deep illness. *Families, Systems, & Health*, *16*(3), 197–212. https://doi.org/10.1037/h0089849

Fuks, A. (2018). Joining the club. *Perspectives in Biology and Medicine*, *61*(2), 279–293.

Fuks, A., Brawer, J., & Boudreau, J. D. (2012). The foundation of physicianship. *Perspectives in Biology and Medicine*, *55*(1), 114–126.

George, D. R. (2010). Overcoming the social death of dementia through language. *The Lancet*, *376*(9741), 586–587.

George, D. R., & Whitehouse, P. J. (2014). The war (on terror) on Alzheimer's. *Dementia*, *13*(1), 120–130.

George, D. R., Whitehouse, E. R., & Whitehouse, P. J. (2016). Asking more of our metaphors: Narrative strategies to end the "war on Alzheimer's" and humanize cognitive aging. *The American Journal of Bioethics*, *16*(10), 22–24.

Geuter, S., Koban, L., & Wager, T. D. (2017). The cognitive neuroscience of placebo effects: Concepts, predictions, and physiology. *Annual Review of Neuroscience*, *40*, 167–188.

Gould, S. J. (1991). The median is not the message. *Bully for Brontosaurus*, 473–477.

Gracely, R. H., Dubner, R., Deeter, W. R., & Wolskee, P. J. (1985). Clinicians' expectations influence placebo analgesia. *Lancet*, *1*(8419), 43.

Grondin, J. (2003). *The philosophy of Gadamer* (K. Plant, Trans.). McGill-Queens University Press.

Hacking, I. (1995). The looping effects of human kinds. In D. Sperber, D. Premack, & A. J. Premack (Eds.), *Causal cognition: A multidisciplinary debate* (pp. 351–394). Clarendon Press/Oxford University Press.

Hacking, I. (2007). Kinds of people: Moving targets. *Proceedings of the British Academy*, *151*, 285–318.

Harper, L. C. (2020). *On vanishing: Mortality, dementia, and what it means to disappear.* Catapult.

Hauser, D. J., & Schwarz, N. (2015). The war on prevention: Bellicose cancer metaphors hurt (some) prevention intentions. *Personality and Social Psychology Bulletin*, *41*(1), 66–77. https://doi.org/10.1177/0146167214557006

Hauser, D. J., & Schwarz, N. (2020). The war on prevention II: Battle metaphors undermine cancer treatment and prevention and do not increase vigilance. *Health Communication*, *35*(13), 1698–1704. https://doi.org/10.1080/10410236.2019.1663465

Hawkins, A. (1984). Two pathographies: A study in illness and literature. *The Journal of Medicine and Philosophy: A Forum for Bioethics and Philosophy of Medicine*, *9*(3), 231–252.

Hawkins, A. H. (1990). A change of heart: The paradigm of regeneration in medical and religious narrative. *Perspectives in Biology and Medicine*, *33*(4), 547–559.

Hawkins, A. H. (1999). *Reconstructing illness: Studies in pathography* (2nd ed.). Purdue University Press.

Haygarth, J. (1800). *Of the imagination: as a cause and as a cure of disorders of the body; exemplified by fictitious tractors, and epidemical convulsions.* R. Cruttwell.

Heritage, J., Robinson, J., Elliott, M., Beckett, M., & Wilkes, M. (2007). Reducing patients' unmet concerns in primary care: The difference one word can make. *Journal of General Internal Medicine, 22*(10), 1429–1433. https://doi.org/10.1007/s11606-007-0279-0

Herrett, E., Williamson, E., Brack, K., Beaumont, D., Perkins, A., Thayne, A., … Smeeth, L. (2021). Statin treatment and muscle symptoms: series of randomised, placebo controlled n-of-1 trials. *BMJ, 372,* n135. doi:10.1136/bmj.n135

Hoenemeyer, T. W., Kaptchuk, T. J., Mehta, T. S., & Fontaine, K. R. (2018). Open-label placebo treatment for cancer-related fatigue: A randomized-controlled clinical trial. *Scientific Reports, 8*(1), 1–8.

Hoffman, J. (2008, June 1). When thumbs up is no comfort. *New York Times.* https://www.nytimes.com/2008/06/01/health/01stoical.html?searchResultPosition=1

Houston, W. R. (1938). The doctor himself as a therapeutic agent. *Annals of Internal Medicine, 11*(8), 1416–1425. https://doi.org/10.7326/0003-4819-11-8-1416

Howe, L. C., Goyer, J. P., & Crum, A. J. (2017). Harnessing the placebo effect: Exploring the influence of physician characteristics on placebo response. *Health Psychology, 36*(11), 1074–1082. https://doi.org/10.1037/hea0000499

Hu, J. (2020, February 4). *The panic over Chinese people doesn't come from the coronavirus.* https://slate.com/technology/2020/02/coronavirus-panic-racist-profiling-asians.html

Hudson, M. M., & Morton, R. S. (1996). Fracastoro and syphilis: 500 years on. *The Lancet, 348*(9040), 1495–1496.

Ishikawa, H., Hashimoto, H., & Kiuchi, T. (2013). The evolving concept of "patient-centeredness" in patient–physician communication research. *Social Science & Medicine, 96,* 147–153. https://doi.org/https://doi.org/10.1016/j.socscimed.2013.07.026

Jackson, S. W. (1992). The listening healer in the history of psychological healing. *American Journal of Psychiatry, 149,* 1623–1632.

Jacobs, L. (1999). Yetzer Ha-Tov and Yetzer Ha-Ra. In *A concise companion to the Jewish religion.* Oxford University Press. https://www.oxfordreference.com/view/10.1093/acref/9780192800886.001.0001/acref-9780192800886-e-773

Jagosh, J., Boudreau, J. D., Steinert, Y., MacDonald, M. E., & Ingram, L. (2011). The importance of physician listening from the patients' perspective: Enhancing diagnosis, healing, and the doctor patient relationship. *Patient Education and Counseling, 85*(3), 369–374. https://doi.org/10.1016/j.pec.2011.01.028

Jewson, N. D. (1974). Medical knowledge and the patronage system in 18th century England. *Sociology, 8*(3), 369–385.

Jewson, N. D. (1976). The disappearance of the sick-man from medical cosmology, 1770–1870. *Sociology, 10*(2), 225–244. https://doi.org/10.1177/003803857601000202

Johnson, A. H., Brock, C. D., & Zacarias, A. (2014). The legacy of Michael Balint. *The International Journal of Psychiatry in Medicine, 47*(3), 175–192.

Kalanthroff, E., Aslan, C., & Dar, R. (2017). Washing away your sins will set your mind free: Physical cleansing modulates the effect of threatened morality on executive control. *Cognition and Emotion, 31*(1), 185–192.

Kamenica, E., Naclerio, R., & Malani, A. (2013). Advertisements impact the physiological efficacy of a branded drug. *Proceedings of the National Academy of Sciences of the United States of America, 110*(32), 12931–12935.

Kaptchuk, T. J. (2011). Placebo studies and ritual theory: A comparative analysis of Navajo, acupuncture and biomedical healing. *Philosophical Transactions of the Royal Society B: Biological Sciences, 366*(1572), 1849–1858.

Kaptchuk, T. J. (2018). Open-label placebo: Reflections on a research agenda. *Perspectives in Biology and Medicine, 61*(3), 311–334.

Kaptchuk, T. J., Kelley, J. M., Conboy, L. A., Davis, R. B., Kerr, C. E., Jacobson, E. E., Kirsch, I., Schyner, R. N., Nam, B. H., Nguyen, L. T., Park, M., Rivers, A. L., McManus, C., Kokkotou, E., Drossman, D. A., Goldman, P., & Lembo, A. J. (2008). Components of placebo effect: Randomised controlled trial in patients with irritable bowel syndrome. *BMJ, 336*(7651), 999–1003.

King, D. B. (1915). *A scheme for dealing with tuberculosis persists in the County of London: Its application to other cities with some observations on the campaign against tuberculosis.* John Bale, Sons and Danielsson, Ltd.

Kisner, J. (2020). Reiki can't possibly work. So why does it? *The Atlantic*, April. https://www.the-atlantic.com/magazine/archive/2020/04/reiki-cant-possibly-work-so-why-does-it/606808/

Kleinman, A., & Becker, A. E. (1998). "Sociosomatics": The contributions of anthropology to psychosomatic medicine. *Psychosomatic Medicine, 60*(4), 389–393.

Lakoff, G., & Johnson, M. (1980). Conceptual metaphor in everyday language. *The Journal of Philosophy, 77*(8), 453–486. https://doi.org/10.2307/2025464

Latour, B. (1988). *The Pasteurization of France.* Harvard University Press.

Lerner, B. H. (1998). Fighting the war on breast cancer: Debates over early detection, 1945 to the present. *Annals of Internal Medicine, 129*(1), 74–78. https://doi.org/10.7326/0003-4819-129-1-199807010-00028

Levenstein, J. H., McCracken, E. C., McWhinney, I. R., Stewart, M. A., & Brown, J. B. (1986). The patient-centred clinical method. 1. A model for the doctor–patient interaction in family medicine. *Family Practice, 3*(1), 24–30.

Levine, J. D., & Gordon, N. C. (1984). Influence of the method of drug administration on analgesic response. *Nature, 312*(5996), 755–756.

Mackenzie, J. N. (1886). The production of the so-called "rose cold" by means of an artifical rose, with remarks and historical notes. *The American Journal of the Medical Sciences (1827–1924), 91*(181), 45.

May, W. F. (2000). *The physician's covenant: Images of the healer in medical ethics* (2nd ed.). John Knox Press.

Miller, F. G., & Colloca, L. (2010). Semiotics and the placebo effect. *Perspectives in Biology and Medicine, 53*(4), 509–516.

Miller, F. G., Colloca, L., & Kaptchuk, T. J. (2009). The placebo effect: Illness and interpersonal healing. *Perspectives in Biology and Medicine, 52*(4), 518–539.

Mishler, E. G. (1984). *The discourse of medicine: Dialectics of medical interviews.* Ablex Publishing Corporation.

Moerman, D. E. (2002). Explanatory mechanisms for placebo effects: Cultural influences and the meaning response. In H. Guess, L. Engel, A. Kleinman, & J. Kusek (Eds.), *The science of the placebo: Toward an interdisciplinary research agenda* (pp. 77–107). BMJ Books.

Moerman, D. E. (2013). Against the "placebo effect": A personal point of view. *Complementary Therapies in Medicine, 21*(2), 125–130.

Mol, A. (2008). *The logic of care: Health and the problem of patient choice.* Routledge.

Montgomery, S. L. (1996). *The scientific voice.* Guilford Press.

Moore, M., & Solomon, H. C. (1935). Joseph Grünpeck and his Neat Treatise (1496) on the French Evil: A translation with a biographical note. *The British Journal of Venereal Diseases, 11*(1), 1–27. https://doi.org/10.1136/sti.11.1.1

Mullan, F. (1985). Seasons of survival: Reflections of a physician with cancer. *New England Journal of Medicine, 313*(4), 270–273.

Mutter, J. (2018). Neglected in the house of medicine. *The Hedgehog Review, 20*(3), 46–56.

Nie, J-B., Gilbertson, A., de Roubaix, M., Staunton, C., van Niekerk, A., Tucker, J. D., & Rennie, S. (2016). Healing without waging war: Beyond military metaphors in medicine and HIV cure research. *American Journal of Bioethics, 16*(10), 3–11.

Niebyl, P. (1982). Commentary. In L. G. Stevenson (Ed.), *A celebration of medical history: The fiftieth anniversary of the Institute of the History of Medicine and the Welch Medical Library* (pp. 154–156). Johns Hopkins University Press.

Nowak, H., Zech, N., Asmussen, S., Rahmel, T., Tryba, M., Oprea, G., Grause, L., Schork, K., Moeller, M., Loeser, J., Gyarmati, K., Mittler, C., Saller, T., Zagler, A., Lutz, K., Adamzik, M., & Hansen, E. (2020). Effect of therapeutic suggestions during general anaesthesia on postoperative pain and opioid use: multicentre randomised controlled trial. *BMJ, 371*, m4284. https://doi.org/10.1136/bmj.m4284

Nutton, V. (1985). Murders and miracles: Lay attitudes towards medicine in classical antiquity. In R. Porter (Ed.), *Patients and practitioners: Lay perceptions of medicine in pre-industrial society* (pp. 23–53). Cambridge University Press.

O'Shea, B. A., Watson, D. G., Brown, G. D., & Fincher, C. L. (2020). Infectious disease prevalence, not race exposure, predicts both implicit and explicit racial prejudice across the United States. *Social Psychological and Personality Science, 11*(3), 345–355.

Ospina, N. S., Phillips, K. A., Rodriguez-Gutierrez, R., Castaneda-Guarderas, A., Gionfriddo, M. R., Branda, M. E., & Montori, V. M. (2019). Eliciting the patient's agenda—Secondary analysis of recorded clinical encounters. *Journal of General Internal Medicine, 34*(1), 36–40.

Otis, L. (1999). *Membranes: Metaphors of invasion in nineteenth-century literature.* John Hopkins University Press.

Pagel, W. (1972). Van Helmont's concept of disease—To be or not to be? The influence of Paracelsus. *Bulletin of the History of Medicine, 46*(5), 419–454.

Paracelsus, & Weeks, A. (Ed.). (2008). *Paracelsus (Theophrastus Bombastus von Hohenheim, 1493–1541): Essential theoretical writings.* Brill.

Park, R. C., Kovera, M. B., & Penrod, S. D. (1992). Jurors' perceptions of eyewitness and hearsay evidence. *Minnesota Law Review, 76,* 703.

Park, L. C., & Covi, L. (1965). Nonblind placebo trial: An exploration of neurotic patients' responses to placebo when its inert content is disclosed. *Archives of General Psychiatry, 12*(4), 336–345.

Pellegrini, I., Rapti, M., Extra, J. M., Petri-Cal, A., Apostolidis, T., Ferrero, J. M., Batchelot, T., Viens, P., Julian-Reynier, C., & Bertucci, F. (2012). Tailored chemotherapy based on tumour gene expression analysis: Breast cancer patients' misinterpretations and positive attitudes. *European Journal of Cancer Care, 21*(2), 242–250.

Penson, R. T., Schapira, L., Daniels, K. J., Chabner, B. A., & Lynch, T. J., Jr. (2004). Cancer as metaphor. *The Oncologist, 9*(6), 708–716.

Perkins, W., Hill, R., & de Bèze, T. (1612). *A golden chaine.* Universitie of Cambridge.

Perrault, S., & O'Keefe, M. M. (2016). Journeys as shared human experiences. *The American Journal of Bioethics, 16*(10), 13–15.

Phillips, D. P., Liu, G. C., Kwok, K., Jarvinen, J. R., Zhang, W., & Abramson, I. S. (2001). The Hound of the Baskervilles effect: Natural experiment on the influence of psychological stress on timing of death. *BMJ, 323*(7327), 1443–1446.

Phillips, T. G., & Hickner, J. (2005). Calling acute bronchitis a chest cold may improve patient satisfaction with appropriate antibiotic use. *Journal of the American Board of Family Practice, 18*(6), 459–463. https://doi.org/10.3122/jabfm.18.6.459

Pollio, H. R., Smith, M. K., & Pollio, M. R. (1990). Figurative language and cognitive psychology. *Language and Cognitive Processes, 5*(2), 141–167.

Qin, A., Myers, S., & Yu., E. (2020, February 6). China tightens Wuhan lockdown in 'wartime' battle with coronavirus. *New York Times.* https://www.nytimes.com/2020/02/06/world/asia/coronavirus-china-wuhan-quarantine.html?searchResultPosition=1

Qiu, C., Xu, W., & Fratiglioni, L. (2010). Vascular and psychosocial factors in Alzheimer's disease: Epidemiological evidence toward intervention. *Journal of Alzheimer's Disease, 20*(3), 689–697.

Quincy, J. (1811). *The American medical lexicon: On the plan of Quincy's lexicon physico-medicum: With many retrenchments, additions, and improvements.* T. and J. Swords.

Rather, L. J. (1982). On the source and development of metaphorical language in the history of Western medicine. In L. G. Stevenson (Ed.), *A celebration of medical history: The fiftieth anniversary of the Institute of the History of Medicine and the Welch Medical Library* (pp. 135–153). Johns Hopkins University Press.

Rather, L. J., & Frerichs, J. B. (1972). On the use of military metaphor in Western medical literature: The bellum contra morbum of Thomas Campanella (1568–1639). *Clio Medica, 7*(3), 201–208.

Rawcliffe, C. (2006). *Leprosy in medieval England.* Boydell Press.

Reisfield, G. M., & Wilson, G. R. (2004). Use of metaphor in the discourse on cancer. *Journal of Clinical Oncology, 22*(19), 4024–4027.

Richardson, J. (2012). *Heidegger* (Ser. Routledge philosophers). Routledge.

Romer, A. L. (1994). *Healing and curing: A psychological exploration of patient–doctor relationships through the experiences of third-year medical students* [9510122, Harvard University]. ProQuest Dissertations & Theses Global.

Rosenberg, C. E. (1987). *The cholera years: The United States in 1832, 1849, and 1866.* University of Chicago Press.

Rosenberg, C. E. (2002). The tyranny of diagnosis: Specific entities and individual experience. *Milbank Quarterly, 80*(2), 237–260.

Ross, J. W. (1989). The militarization of disease: Do we really want a war on AIDS? *Soundings, 71*(1), 39–58.

Ryan, C., & Ryan, K. M. (1979). *A private battle.* Simon and Schuster.

Salmon, P., & Hall, G. M. (2003). Patient empowerment and control: A psychological discourse in the service of medicine. *Social Science & Medicine, 57*(10), 1969–1980.

Salmon, P., & Hall, G. M. (2004). Patient empowerment or the emperor's new clothes. *Journal of the Royal Society of Medicine, 97*(2), 53–56.

Salmon, P., & Young, B. (2017). A new paradigm for clinical communication: Critical review of literature in cancer care. *Medical Education, 51*(3), 258–268.

Saraga, M., Boudreau, D., & Fuks, A. (2019a). An empirical and philosophical exploration of clinical practice. *Philosophy, Ethics, and Humanities in Medicine, 14*(1), 1–11.

Saraga, M., Boudreau, D., & Fuks, A. (2019b). Engagement and practical wisdom in clinical practice: A phenomenological study. *Medicine, Health Care and Philosophy, 22*(1), 41–52. https://doi.org/10.1007/s11019-018-9838-x

Saraga, M., Fuks, A., & Boudreau, J. D. (2014). George Engel's epistemology of clinical practice. *Perspectives in Biology and Medicine, 57*(4), 482–494.

Schei, E., Fuks, A., & Boudreau, J. D. (2019). Reflection in medical education: Intellectual humility, discovery, and know-how. *Medicine, Health Care and Philosophy, 22*(2), 167–178.

Schultz-Schultzenstein, K. H. (1844). *Lehrbuch der allgemeinen Krankheitslehre* (Vol. 1). Hirschwald.

Scott, J. G., Cohen, D., Cicco-Bloom, B., Miller, W. L., Stange, K. C., & Crabtree, B. F. (2008). Understanding healing relationships in primary care. *Annals of Family Medicine, 6*(4), 315–322.

Segal, J. Z. (2005). *Health and the rhetoric of medicine.* SIU Press.

Segal, J. Z. (2019). Ageism and rhetoric. In A. Bleakley (Ed.), *Routledge handbook of the medical humanities* (pp. 163–175). Routledge.

Semino, E., Demjén, Z., Demmen, J., Koller, V., Payne, S., Hardie, A., & Rayson, P. (2017). The online use of violence and journey metaphors by patients with cancer, as compared with health professionals: A mixed methods study. *BMJ Supportive & Palliative Care, 7*(1), 60–66. https://doi.org/10.1136/bmjspcare-2014-000785

Simpson, S. H., Eurich, D. T., Majumdar, S. R., Padwal, R. S., Tsuyuki, R. T., Varney, J., & Johnson, J. A. (2006). A meta-analysis of the association between adherence to drug therapy and mortality. *BMJ, 333*(7557), 15.

Slobod, D., & Fuks, A. (2012). Military metaphors and friendly fire. *CMAJ, 184*(1), 144.

Smith, A. D. (2019). *Notes from the field.* Anchor.

Snævarr. S. (2010). *Metaphors, narratives, emotions: Their interplay and impact* (Series Consciousness, Literature & The Arts, 24). Rodopi.

Sontag, S. (1978). *Illness as metaphor.* Farrar, Straus and Giroux.

Spiro, H. (2009). Commentary: The practice of empathy, *Academic Medicine, 84*(9), 1177–1179. https://doi:10.1097/ACM.0b013e3181b18934

Stibbe, A. (1996). The metaphorical construction of illness in Chinese culture. *Journal of Asian Pacific Communication, 7,* 177–188.

Stiefel, F., & Bourquin, C. (2019). Moving toward the next generation of communication training in oncology: The relevance of findings from qualitative research. *European Journal of Cancer Care, 28,* e13149. https://doi.org/10.1111/ecc.13149

Strout, E. (2019). *Olive, again.* Random House.

Suchman, A. L., & Matthews, D. A. (1988). What makes the patient–doctor relationship therapeutic? Exploring the connexional dimension of medical care. *Annals of Internal Medicine, 108*(1), 125–130. https://doi.org/10.7326/0003-4819-108-1-125

Sydenham, T., Locke, J., & Meynell, G. G. (1991). *Thomas Sydenham's observations medicae (London, 1676) and his medical observations, (manuscript 572 of the Royal College of Physicians of London); with new transcripts of related Locke mss. in the Bodleian Library.* Winterdown Books.

Tauber, A. I. (2016). Immunity in context: Science and society in dialogue. *THEORIA. An International Journal for Theory, History and Foundations of Science, 31*(2), 207–224.

Taylor, C. (2016). *The language animal: The full shape of the human linguistic capacity.* Belknap Press of Harvard University Press.

Temkin, O. (1977). *The double face of Janus and other essays in the history of medicine.* Johns Hopkins University Press.

Thomas, K. B. (1987). General practice consultations: Is there any point in being positive? *British Medical Journal Clinical Research Education, 294*(6581), 1200–1202.

Tomes, N. (1990). *The gospel of germs: Men, women, and the microbe in American life.* Harvard University Press.

Virchow, R. (1847). Ueber die Reform der pathologischen und therapeutischen Anschauungen durch die mikroskopischen Untersuchungen. *Archiv für pathologische Anatomie und Physiologie und für klinische Medicin, 1*(2), 207–255. https://doi.org/10.1007/BF01975870

Virchow, R. (1885). Special article: The battle of cells and bacteria. *JAMA, V*(8), 216–220.

Wear, A. (1985). Puritan perceptions of illness in seventeenth century England. In R. Porter (Ed.), *Patients and practitioners: Lay perceptions of medicine in pre-industrial society* (pp. 55–99). Cambridge University Press.

Williams, K. N., Herman, R., Gajewski, B., & Wilson, K. (2009). Elderspeak communication: Impact on dementia care. *American Journal of Alzheimer's Disease & Other Dementia, 24*(1), 11–20. https://doi.org/10.1177/1533317508318472

Woolf, V. (1930). *On being ill.* Hogarth Press.

Zhong, C-B., & Liljenquist, K. A. (2006). Washing away your sins: Threatened morality and physical cleansing. *Science, 313*(5792), 1451–1452.

Zinsser, H. (1934). *Rats, lice and history.* Little & Brown.

Zulman, D. M., Haverfield, M. C., Shaw, J. G., Brown-Johnson, C. G., Schwartz, R., Tierney, A. A., Zionts, D. L., Safaeinili, N., Fischer, M., Thadaney Israni, S., Asch, S. M., & Verghese, A. (2020). Practices to foster physician presence and connection with patients in the clinical encounter. *JAMA, 323*(1), 70–81. https://doi.org/10.1001/jama.2019.19003

Index

For the benefit of digital users, indexed terms that span two pages (e.g., 52–53) may, on occasion, appear on only one of those pages.

Tables are indicated by *t* following the page number.

ageism, 32
agency
    journey metaphor, 115–18
    patient-directed care, 57–58, 166–68
    patient versus disease model, 55–57
    physician as mercenary model, 57–58
AI (artificial intelligence), 93–94
AIDS, 86, 99
allegory, 71–72, 73–74
allergic skin reactions, placebo interventions
        for, 143–44
alterity, 185–86
Alzheimer's disease, 109–10, 111–12
analgesic administration, placebo interventions
        for, 144–45, 148–49, 155–56
anchor point, 176–77
ancient Greece, understanding of disease in, 70
Annas, G., 113–14
antibiotics, 21
any-, 21
Aris's Birmingham Gazette, 66
Armstrong, L., 100–1
artificial intelligence (AI), 93–94
associative learning, 149–51, 152–53
athletic fighter, 100–1
attentive listening, 128–30
autonomy of patients, 166–68

bacteria
    associated with dirt and pollution, 72
    early war metaphors related to, 64–66
    effect of environment on growth of, 80
    germ theory, 63–64
balance, 114–15
Balint, M., 123, 145–46, 155, 166, 168–69, 182–83
battle metaphors. *See* war metaphors
Baziak, A. T., 79–80
Becker, C., 74
bellum contra morbum, 67–68
Benedetti, F., 155
biological metaphors, 37–38
biopsychosocial model, 163–65
blame
    assigning to patients, 17–19

autonomy and empowerment, effects of, 167–68
    in doctor versus disease model, 53–54
    during epidemics, 85–86
    factors affecting, 82–85
    genetics and, 93–94
    in patient versus disease model, 55–56
    in physician as mercenary model, 58
    sanitarian movements and, 88
BODY IS A MACHINE metaphor, 38, 41–42
Boerhaave, H., 66–67, 68–69
Boudreau, D., 123
boundaries, trespassing, 173–74
Bourquin, C., 171–72
Brissot, P., 66–68
Broyard, A., 117–18, 179

Campanella, T., 67–68
cancer
    concealment of diagnosis, 57
    doctor reactions to end-of-life care, 54
    early detection and prevention, 18–19
    early ideas on sin as cause of, 68
    effect of war metaphors on patients, 168
    as enemy, 59–60
    framing, examples of, 22
    journey metaphor, 116–17
    pathography, war metaphors in, 95–99
    sense of guilt associated with, 82–83
    survivors, discussion of term, 29–32
    war metaphors related to, 50, 90
Canguilhem, G., 114–15
Cannon, W., 114–15
Cassell, E., 181
CBME (competency-based medical
        education), 10–11
Centers for Disease Control and Prevention
        (CDC), 51–52
chaos, 118–19, 175–76
chief complaint, use of phrase, 18
children, use of metaphors with, 117–18
Chinese Americans, mortality rates from heart
        disease among, 152
Chochinov, H., 186
Cholera Years, The (Rosenberg), 84–85

Christianity
  allegory, 72–74
  moral nature of disease, 68–69
  priests, parallels between physicians and, 92
  Psychomachia, 70–72
chronic traumatic encephalopathy, 110–11
cleanliness, 84–85
  sanitarian movements, 87–89
clinical communication, 28–29
clinical distance, 15
clinical encounter
  engagement in, 8–9
  insensitivity in use of metaphors, 100–1
  learning in, 9
  modalities of clinical work, 9–10
  tailored relationships, 183–85
clinical listening, 127–32
  informational, 127–28
  maieutic, 130–32, 133.
  relational, 128–30
  tailored responsiveness, 185
  transactional, 128
clinical presence, 170–72, 185
clinical work
  metaphors in, 44–45
  modalities of, 9–10
cognitive bias, 21–22
cognitive metaphors, 34–35
Cohn, C., 42–44
collaborative framing, 161–63
Colloca, L., 153–54
collusion of anonymity, 168–69
colors, linguistic relativity and, 23–24
commanders, physicians as, 101–3
competency-based medical education (CBME), 10–11
complaints, patient, 18
complementary and alternative medicine, 144
compliance, patient, 18
computer-assisted medicine, 11
CONTAINER source domain, 35–36, 38–39
COVID-19 pandemic
  ecological metaphors related to, 114
  physician-patient communication during, 183
  social determinants, 110–11
  war metaphors related to, 85–86, 120, 162
craftmanship, 191
critical listening, 126
Crusades, 73–74
cultural associative learning, 151, 152
culture, influence on metaphors, 38, 39–41, 42
curing versus healing, 181

defensive listening, 127
dementia, 20–21, 109–10, 111–12
Dentan, R. K., 79–80

descriptive linguistic form, 3, 4, 6–8
detachment, 8–9, 15
diagnosis, 57, 77–80
diamonds, 158
dirt, role in disease, 72–74
  sanitarian movements, 87–89
"Disappearance of the Sick-Man from Medical
  Cosmology, The" (Jewson), 82
disease
  diagnosis of, 77–80
  dirt and sins associated with, 72–74
  doctor versus, 51–55
  as enemy of society, 58–60
  epidemics, 85–86, 89–90, 114
  germ theory of, 63–64
  guilt and blame for, 82–85
  illness versus, 80–82
  medical luminaries, war metaphors used
    by, 66–68
  moral nature of, 68–69
  patient versus, 55–57
  prevention, 89–91
  sanitarian movements, 87–89
  search for meaning and, 70–72
  therapy, 91–92
Diski, J., 117
disparate attentional anchors, 132–33
doctor as drug, 155, 156–57, 182–83
doctor as placebo, 156–57
doctor–patient relationship. *See* physician-patient
  relationship
doctors. *See* physicians
Donne, J., 69
dopamine, 147–48
Douglas, M., 72
drug trials, placebos in, 141–42
dual discourse of clinical medicine, 135–36, 165
dyadic relationship
  clinical presence, 170–72
  components of, 169
  humility in, 185–87
  tailored relationships, 183–85
dystasis, 114–15

early cancer detection and prevention, 18–19
EBM (evidence-based medicine), 12–13
ecological metaphors, 111–12, 113–14
Einfuhlung, 8–9
elderly patients, using infantilizing language
  with, 20–21
electronic health records, 11, 125–26
empathy, 8–9, 28, 131
empowerment of patients, 166–68
end-of-life care, 54, 60
enemy of society, disease as, 58–60

engagement, 8–9
  balancing detachment and, 15
  clinical presence, 170–72, 185
  maieutic listening, 130–32, 177
  testimonies to relational care, 173–77
Engel, G., 163–65, 172
Enlightenment, 74
entailments, metaphoric, 35
epidemics, 85–86, 89–90, 114. *See also* COVID-19
  pandemic
evidence-based medicine (EBM), 12–13
experience, medical, 11

false dichotomy, 134–36
familial expectation to fight, 56–57
fighting physician, 101–3
fighting words, 103–5
figurative linguistic form, 9–10, 34–35, 41, 45, 184
figures of speech, 120–21
Findley, T., 155
Fissell, M., 77, 81–82
fitness of metaphors, 39–41
Fiumara, G., 130–31, 136
Fletcher, A., 71–72
Flexner Report (1910), 163
footing, 13–15
Fowler, F. G., 33–34
Fowler, H. W., 33–34
framework of relationships, 169–70
framing
  cancer survivors, 29–32
  collaborative, 161–63
  diagnosis of disease, 77–80
  general discussion, 21–22
  with metaphors, 41–42
Frank, A., 118–19, 123, 131, 175–76
frequency of metaphors, 39–40, 60–61

Gadamer, H.-G., 6, 9, 136
Galen, 67–68
gendered nouns, 23–24
genomic medicine, 93
George, D., 111–12
germ theory, 63–64
goal confusion, 132–33
Gospel of Germs, The (Tomes), 87–89
Gould, S. J., 152–53
Gracely, R. H., 155–56
Greece, understanding of disease in ancient, 70
Grünpeck von Burckhausen, J., 69
guilt
  autonomy and empowerment, effects of, 167–68
  factors affecting sense of, 82–85
  genetics and, 93–94
  sanitarian movements, 88

Hacking, I., 29, 31
Hall, G. M., 167–68
handwashing, 84
HAPPINESS IS UP metaphor, 37–38
Harper, L. C., 109–10
Hauser, D. J., 90
Hawkins, A. H., 96–99, 103–4, 115–16, 117–18
Haygarth, J., 139, 141–42
healing, concept of, 179–81
healing metaphors
  concept of healing, 179–81
  doctor as drug, 182–83
  general discussion, 187–90
  humility, 185–87
  measured words, 181–82
  physicians and language, 190–91
  tailored relationships, 183–85
HEALTH source domain, 39
heart disease, mortality rates from, 152
Heartsounds (Lear), 98–99
*Heavenly City of the Eighteenth-Century
  Philosophers, The* (Becker), 74
Heidegger, M., 7–8, 136
hermeneutics of clinical practice, 4–9, 134–35
Hippocrates, 139–40
HIV-related illnesses, 113, 117
homeopathic remedies, 144
homeostasis, 38, 114–15
honest work, 173
hope, 169
house of being, language as, 7–9
humanities versus natural sciences, 134–35, 134t
humility, 6, 185–87
humoral model of medicine, 38
hygiene, 72–74, 84–85
  sanitarian movements, 87–89

idiolects, 24–25, 28
illness
  disease versus, 80–82
  journey metaphor, 115–18
  kingdom of the ill, 26–27, 39–40, 55, 115–16
  pathography, 95–99
  in traditional Chinese medicine, 112–13
Illness as Metaphor (Sontag), 39–40, 64
immunology, 64–66, 90–91
incidentaloma, 53
individuality of patients, acknowledging, 169–70
infantilizing language, 20–21
infections, war metaphors related to, 64–66
informational listening, 127–28
informed consent, 141–42
interrogative listening, 127
irritable bowel syndrome, placebo interventions
  for, 143–44

Japanese Americans, mortality rates from heart disease among, 152
jaundice, 25–26
Jewson, N.D., 82
journey, illness as, 115–18
judgmental form of questioning, 127
Just A Medical Student (JAMS), 22–23, 168–69

Kaptchuk, T., 152
ketorolac, 148–49
kingdom of the ill, 26–27, 39–40, 55, 115–16
Kleinman, A., 80–81, 153–54
known, sense of being, 169

labeling, social, 29–32
language. *See also* metaphors; pharmacology of words
    clinical communication, 28–29
    framing, 21–22
    as house of being, 7–9
    infantilizing, 20–21
    influence on metaphors, 42
    Just A Medical Student, 22–23, 168–69
    linguistic relativity, 23–28
    making up people, 29–32
    measured words, 181–82
    physicians and, 190–91
    potency of small words, 21
    reciprocity, 19–20
    registers and footings, 13–15
    reimagining illnesses through new, 110–12
    responsibility and blame, 17–19
    tailored relationships, 183–85
Latour, B., 87
Lear, M., 98–99
Les Microbes: Guerre et Paix (Latour), 87
LESS IS DOWN metaphor, 37–38
Levinas, E., 185–86
Liljenquist, K. A., 84
liminality, 115–16
linguistic interaction, modes of, 3–9
linguistic relativity, 23–28
listening
    clinical, 127–32
    emphasis on speaking versus, 124–25, 136
    false dichotomy, 134–36
    general discussion, 123–26
    goal confusion, 132–33
    in medical education, 137
    modes of, 126–27
    role confusion, 132–33
Lloyd's Weekly London Newspaper, 66
Logic of Care: Health and the Problem of Patient Choice, The (Mol), 166–67

logos versus *legein*, 136
looping effect, 31

magic bubble, creating, 174
making up people, 29–32
mapping metaphors, 35–37
May, W., 102
McKenzie, J., 150
meaning, concept of, 153–54
meaning, search for, 70–72
measured words, 181–82
"Median Isn't the Message, The" (Gould), 152–53
medical education
    language training, 190–91
    listening training, 137
    methodological changes in, 10–11
    world view changed by, 22–23
medical interviews, care with small words in, 21
medical luminaries, war metaphors used by, 66–68
medical students, 22–23, 168–69
mercenary, physician as, 57–58
metaphors. *See also* healing metaphors; war metaphors
    balance and homeostasis, 114–15
    in clinical setting, 44–45
    cognitive, 34–35
    culture and language, influence on, 42
    describing dementia, 109–10
    ecological, 111–12, 113–14
    effect on thought and being, 42–44
    figures of speech, 120–21
    fitness of, 39–41
    framing reality, 41–42
    history of, 34
    illness as journey, 115–18
    mapping, 35–37
    missing, 119–20
    placebo as, 156–57
    quest narrative, 118–19
    reimagining illnesses through, 110–12
    roots of, 37–39
    in traditional Chinese medicine, 112–13
    UNDERSTANDING IS SEEING framework, 33–34, 35–37
Metchnikoff, I., 64–65
metonymy, 44
micro-cultures, linguistic relativity in, 24, 28
military leaders, physicians as, 101–3
military metaphors. *See* war metaphors
Miller, F. G., 153–54, 155
MIND IS A COMPUTER metaphor, 38–39, 41–42
MIND IS A CONTAINER metaphor, 36, 38–39
minister, discussion of term, 92

Modern Health Crusades, 88–89
Moerman, D., 153–54
Mol, A., 166–67, 169–70
Montgomery, S., 64
moral nature of disease, 68–69
MORE IS UP metaphor, 37–38
Mutter, J., 78–79

naloxone, 147, 148–49
narratives of illness
    journey metaphor, 115–18
    loss of focus on, 81–82
    of physicians, 27
    quest narrative, 118–19
National Tuberculosis Association (NTA), 88–89
natural sciences
    versus humanities, 134–35, 134t
    metaphors used in, 40–41
Navajo rituals, 152
"Need for a New Medical Model: A Challenge for
    Biomedicine, The" (Engel), 163–64
negotiation metaphors, 39
New England Journal of Medicine, 113–14
New York Times, 66, 109
Nie, J- B., 113, 117
nocebos, 150–51, 152–54, 187–89
non-compliant patients, 18
NTA (National Tuberculosis Association), 88–89
nuclear defense planners, metaphors used
    by, 42–44
Nutton, V., 70

O'Keefe, M. M., 117
"On Being Ill" (Woolf), 115–16
open/covert placebo research, 144–46, 149
opening questions, 5
open-label placebos, 146–47, 149, 152–53, 154
opioid systems, role in placebo response, 147–49
optimism, 56
orientational metaphors, 37–38
Osler, W., 65–66
Oxford English Dictionary (OED), 33–34, 36–37,
    139–40, 181

pain relief, placebo interventions for, 144–45, 148–
    49, 155–56
palliative care, 54, 60
Paracelsus, 66–67, 68
Parkinson's disease, placebo interventions
    for, 147–48
Pasteur, L., 63–64, 87
pathography, 95–99, 115–18
patient-centered medicine, 9–10, 165–68
patient-directed care, 14–15, 57–58, 166–68

patients. See also physician-patient communication;
        physician-patient relationship
    autonomy and empowerment, effects of, 167–68
    as battleground in doctor versus disease
        model, 52–53
    benefits of war metaphor for, 103–5
    effects of war metaphors on, 168
    illness in, 80–82
    individuality of, acknowledging, 169–70
    infantilizing language, using with, 19–20
    pathography, 95–99, 115–18
    patient versus disease model, 55–57
    reciprocity from, 19–20
    responsibility and blame placed on, 17–19
Pavlovian conditioning, 149
Penson, R. T., 117–18
perceptual metaphors, 37–38
Perkins, William, 69
Perrault, S., 117, 120
personal associative learning, 150
personal behavior, effect on disease, 84
personalized medicine, 93
personal responsibility, 174
Peter of Abano, 67
Pettenkofer, M. J., 80
pharmacology of words
    associative learning, 149–51
    clinical benefits of placebos, 142–47
    modes of elicitation, 149–51
    physiological mechanisms of placebos, 147–49
    placebo as metaphor, 156–57
    relational placebo, 155–56
    rituals and social communication, 152–54
physical cleanliness, 84–85
physician-patient communication. See also
        listening; pharmacology of words
    clinical communication, 28–29
    fitness of metaphors, 104–5, 120
    framing, 21–22
    infantilizing language, 20–21
    linguistic relativity, 23–28
    making up people, 29–32
    reciprocity in, 19–20
    responsibility and blame in, 17–19
    small words, power of, 21
physician-patient relationship
    clinical presence, 170–72
    collaborative framing, 161–63
    framework of relationships, 169–70
    JAMS, 22–23, 168–69
    modes of linguistic interaction in, 3–9
    patient-centered medicine, 165–68
    reciprocity in, 19–20
    registers and footings, effect on, 13–15

physician-patient relationship (*cont.*)
  reintroducing patient in medical
    models, 163–65
  shared management of risks, 19
  teams, treatment of patient by, 168–69
  testimonies to relational, 173–77
physicians. *See also* physician-patient
    communication; physician-patient
    relationship
  benefits of placebos linked to, 142–47
  doctor as drug, 155, 156–57, 182–83
  doctor as placebo, 156–57
  doctor versus disease model, 51–55
  historical importance of, 92
  medical luminaries, war metaphors used
    by, 66–68
  narratives of illness of, 27
  physician as mercenary model, 57–58
Physician's Covenant, The (May), 102
placebos
  clinical benefits, 142–47
  in drug trials, 141–42
  effects, 142
  history of, 139–42
  as metaphor, 156–57
  modes of elicitation, 149–51
  open/covert research, 144–46, 149
  open-label, 146–47, 149, 152–53, 154
  physiological mechanisms of, 147–49
  relational placebo, 155–56
  responses, 142
  rituals and social communication, 152–54
pneumonia, 52–53
Pollio, H. R., 39–40
pollution, disease associated with, 72
presence, clinical, 170–72
prevention of disease, 89–91
priests, parallels between physicians and, 92
Private Battle, A (Ryan), 95–99
proceduralists, 102–3
Proust, M., 150
Prudentius, A., 70–72
pseudo-listening, 126
psychological conditioning, 149
Psychomachia (Prudentius), 70–72
purgations, 69
Puritan beliefs about disease, 69

questions, care with small words in, 21
quest narrative, 118–19
quotidian discourse, military metaphors in, 66

racism, epidemics and, 85–86
randomized clinical trials, placebos
  in, 141–42
readiness, 174

reality
  framing by metaphors, 41–42
  metaphors used to distance from, 42–44
reciprocal engagement, 131
reciprocity in care, 19–20
recovery, 114–15
reflective attention to language, 19–20
registers, 13–15, 24
reified disease, 52–53, 78–80
reimagining illnesses, 110–12
Reisfleld, G. M., 100–1, 116–18
relational care
  clinical presence, 170–72
  components of, 169–70
  humility in, 185–87
  tailored relationships, 183–85
  testimonies to, 173–77
relational listening, 128–30
relational placebo, 155–56
relational understanding, 169
resilience of military metaphors
  fighting physician, 101–3
  fighting words, 103–5
  overview, 95
  A Private Battle (Ryan), 95–99
  sports metaphors, 100–1
responsibility, assignment of
  autonomy and empowerment, effects of, 167–68
  in doctor versus disease model, 53–54
  factors affecting, 82–85
  to patients, 17–19
  in patient versus disease model, 55–56
  in physician as mercenary model, 58
restitution, 118–19
rhetorical divergence, 133
rheumatoid arthritis, placebo interventions
  for, 144
risks, shared management of, 19
rites of passage, 115–16
rituals, 152–54
robots, 93–94
role confusion, 132–33
role models, power of, 150–51
Romer, A., 22–23
roots of metaphors, 37–39
Rosenberg, C., 79–80, 84–85
Ross, J. W., 86
Ryan, C., 95–99

Sacks, O., 115–16
SADNESS IS DOWN metaphor, 37–38
Salmon, P., 167–68
sanitarian movements, 87–89
Saraga, M., 164, 172
Schultz, C. H., 64
Schwarz, N., 90

Scott, J., 131–32, 169
search for meaning, 70–72
seasonal variation of metaphors, 39
seeing, metaphors related to, 33–34
Segal, J., 32
selective breeding, metaphoric extensions
    of, 40–41
self-directed medical care, 57–58
semiosis, 25–26
sense of being known, 169
shared mind, 179
shock, as reaction to illness, 175
Simpson, S., 154
sin, relatedness of disease and
    moral nature of disease, 68–69
    Psychomachia, 70–72
small words, power of, 21
Smith, A. D., 131
social associative learning, 150–51
social communication, 152–54
social determinants of health, 83–84,
    110–12, 120
social expectation to fight, 56–57
social labeling, 29–32
social media, effect on communication, 125
social probe, 127
societal trends, effect on clinical relationship, 11
sociolects, 24–27, 28
sociosomatics, 153–54
some-, 21
Sontag, S., 25–26, 29–30, 39–40, 57, 64
sources of war metaphors
    cultural change and stability, 74
    dirt and sins associated with disease, 72–74
    disease and search for meaning, 70–72
    early sources of, 64–66
    evolving strands of, 75
    medical luminaries, 66–68
    moral nature of disease, 68–69
    Pasteur's germ theory, 63–64
    Psychomachia, 70–72
    quotidian discourse, 66
spatially directed expectancy, 147
speaking, imbalance between listening and, 124–
    25, 136
Spiro, H., 131
sports metaphors, 100–1
Stibbe, A., 112
Stiefel, F., 171–72
Strout, E., 161
survivors of cancer, 29–32
Sydenham, T., 66–67, 68
syphilis, 69, 85

tailored relationships, 183–85
Tauber, A., 90–91

taxonomy of diseases, 78–80
Taylor, C., 7–8
TCM (traditional Chinese medicine), 112–13
teams, treatment of patient by, 168–69
technology, effect on communication, 125
Temkin, O., 72
Ten Commandments for Keeping Baby Well, The
    (pamphlet), 88
testimonies to relational, 173–77
therapy, 91–92, 93–94
thought and being, effect of metaphors on, 42–44
time, 13, 171
Tomes, N., 87–89
traditional Chinese medicine (TCM), 112–13
training in listening, 137
transactional listening, 128
transformative symbolic structures, 42
treatment, 91–92
trespassing boundaries, 173–74
tropes of war, 72–73, 73t
trust, 169
tuberculosis, 88–89
Turner, V., 115–16

UNDERSTANDING IS SEEING framework,
    33–34, 35–37

vaccinations, 17–18
Vico, G., 135–36
violence metaphors, 60
Virchow, R., 64–66
virus metaphors, 119–20
VISUAL FIELD IS A CONTAINER
    metaphor, 35–36
visual metaphors, 37–38
von Helmont, J. B., 66–67, 68

war metaphors. *See also* sources of war metaphors
    battle and violence metaphors, 60
    collaborative framing versus, 161–63
    disease as enemy of society, 58–60
    doctor versus disease model, 51–55
    effect on cancer patients, 168
    effect on disease prevention, 89–91
    effect on therapy, 91–92
    niche for, 188–89
    patient versus disease model, 55–57
    physician as mercenary model, 57–58
    prevalence of, 49–51
    tropes of war, 72–73, 73t
    in wartime, 60–61
"When Thumbs Up is No Comfort" (*New York
    Times*), 56
Whorf-Sapir effect, 23–25
Wilson, G. R., 100–1, 117–18
Wittgenstein, L., 193

Women's Field Army, The, 50
Woolf, V., 24–25, 115–16
world view
    illness, effect on, 26–27
    metaphoric language, effect on, 42–44
writing, frequency of metaphors in, 39–40

xenophobia, 85–86

Young, B., 167–68

Zhong, C- B., 84
Zinsser, H., 65–66